Unravelling the Layers of Chronic Illness and Loneliness

Sophie Lewis · Karen Willis ·
Lorraine Smith ·
Maja Lindegaard Moensted ·
Marika Franklin · Leslie Dubbin ·
Anne Rogers

Unravelling the Layers of Chronic Illness and Loneliness

A Social Perspective

palgrave
macmillan

Sophie Lewis
Sydney School of Health Sciences
The University of Sydney
Camperdown, NSW, Australia

Lorraine Smith
Sydney School of Pharmacy
The University of Sydney
Camperdown, NSW, Australia

Marika Franklin
Sydney School of Health Sciences
The University of Sydney
Camperdown, NSW, Australia

Anne Rogers
Faculty of Health Sciences
University of Southampton
Southampton, UK

Karen Willis
Institute for Health and Sport
Victoria University
Melbourne, VIC, Australia

Maja Lindegaard Moensted
Sydney School of Health Sciences
The University of Sydney
Camperdown, NSW, Australia

Leslie Dubbin
School of Nursing
University of California, San Francisco
San Francisco, CA, USA

ISBN 978-981-96-7908-9 ISBN 978-981-96-7909-6 (eBook)
https://doi.org/10.1007/978-981-96-7909-6

Cover illustration: Justin Paget

This Palgrave Macmillan imprint is published by the registered company Springer Nature Singapore Pte Ltd.
The registered company address is: 152 Beach Road, #21-01/04 Gateway East, Singapore 189721, Singapore

Acknowledgement of Country

We acknowledge that this research was conducted on the unceded lands of the Gadigal people of the Eora nation and the Wurundjeri and Wathaurong peoples of the Kulin nation. We pay our respects to their Elders past and present.

The original version of the book has been revised. A correction to this book can be found at https://doi.org/10.1007/978-981-96-7909-6

Acknowledgements We express our gratitude to all those who took part in our research study, who so generously gave of their time and shared their experiences with us. We are grateful to those who provided assistance with recruitment of participants to this study, including MS Australia, Uniting NSW, Carers NSW, and Carers WA. We thank Professor Natasha Smallwood, Professor of Respiratory Medicine, Monash University and Head, Breathlessness and Advanced Respiratory Disease Clinic, Alfred Hospital Melbourne for her assistance with recruitment and her clinician expertise.

Our appreciation is also extended to our research assistants, Dr Melissa Cheung, Alana Munro and Kristina Sokolova whose attention to detail and dedication contributed to the success of this project.

This book is based on a research study funded by an Australian Research Council (ARC) Discovery Project Grant [DP200101872]. We are grateful for their recognition of the importance of understanding the intersection between loneliness and chronic illness.

Competing Interests The authors have no competing interests to declare that are relevant to the content of this manuscript.

Ethics Approval This book reports on findings from a qualitative research study that was performed in line with the principles of the Declaration of Helsinki. Approval was granted by the University of New South Wales Human Research Ethics Committee (June 2020/no. HC200333) and the University of Sydney Human Research Ethics Committee (December 2021/no. 2021/909). All participants provided written or verbal informed consent prior to enrolment in the study.

Contents

About the Authors

Associate Professor Sophie Lewis is a health sociologist in the Faculty of Medicine and Health at the University of Sydney. Her research takes a person-centred approach, focusing on experiences of people living with long-term conditions and the social forces that shape these experiences. Her current research explores loneliness and social connectedness for those living with chronic illness, young people's experiences of growing up with chronic illness, social perspectives on end-of-life care, death and dying, living with incurable cancers, and navigating the complexity of healthcare choices and costs. She is Associate Editor of Health Sociology Review, and co-author of *Experiences of Healthcare Workers During the COVID-19 Pandemic: In Their Own Words* (2022) Routledge (with M Bismark, K Willis and N Smallwood).

Professor Karen Willis is a health sociologist and Professor of Public Health at Victoria University, Melbourne and a research affiliate at the University of Sydney. Her research focuses on the intersections between personal choices and public ideas and discourses. She has examined healthcare choice in relation to private health insurance, how people set goals when self-managing chronic conditions, and the psychosocial impact of COVID-19 on healthcare workers. Recent books include *Experiences of Healthcare Workers During the COVID-19 Pandemic: In Their Own Words* (2022) Routledge (with M Bismark, S Lewis and N Smallwood); *The COVID-19 Crisis: Social Perspectives*, 2021 (edited with D Lupton) Routledge; *Navigating Private and Public Healthcare—Experiences of Patients, Doctors and Policy Makers.*2020, (edited with F Collyer). From 2019 to 2022 she was joint editor-in-chief of *Health Sociology Review.*

Professor Lorraine Smith is a research psychologist in the Faculty of Medicine and Health at the University of Sydney. Her work focuses on patient experiences and self-management of long-term conditions and how patients and health professionals negotiate goal setting. She is a foundation member and past Chair of DIPEx International, an association of qualitative researchers worldwide committed to understanding health and illness experiences globally.

Dr. Maja Lindegaard Moensted is a sociologist and research fellow in the Faculty of Medicine and Health at the University of Sydney. Taking a qualitative approach, her research focuses on developing sociological understandings of the experiences of disadvantaged people in their meeting with welfare institutions. The bulk of her research has been dedicated to improving understandings, policies and practice of how best to support people experiencing disadvantage to thrive and developing innovative, participatory methodologies able to capture different types of knowledge and give voice to people who struggle to participate in traditional data generation methods. A particular research focus is youth disadvantage; the relationship between social connectedness and health; substance use; homelessness and integrated care for highly marginalised consumers. Collectively her research provides insights into the complexity of health and social inequities across different populations and care contexts.

Dr. Marika Franklin is a research fellow and lecturer in the Faculty of Medicine and Health at the University of Sydney and Honorary

Research Fellow at Deakin University. As an interdisciplinary qualitative researcher, her research is situated at the intersection of psychology and sociology. Marika's interests are in the relational aspects of self-management and person-centred care for people living with long-term conditions. Her current research focuses on health and well-being for older migrants and those living with long-term conditions, with specific attention to patient–professional interactions, patient reported outcome measures, self-care, and self-management. Marika is an advocate in the community and policy space, and as a Director for the Multicultural Communities Council of NSW, recently provided evidence for the Inquiry into the prevalence, causes, and impacts of loneliness in New South Wales.

Associate Professor Leslie Dubbin is a health policy researcher in the School of Nursing at the University of California, San Francisco. Her program of research investigates the social and health impacts of public housing renovation and redevelopment, the intersection of place and health, and the ways in which social and racial inequalities manifest throughout the healthcare system.

Professor Anne Rogers is Emeritus Professor of Medical Sociology at the University of Southampton. Her research interests are in the sociological aspects of mental health and illness, self-care and management of long-term conditions, people's experiences of health care, health need and demand for care, and how patients adapt to and incorporate new technologies into their everyday life. Her most recent interests are focused on addressing how social ties and relationships operate in domestic and community settings and act as a conduit for accessing resources and support for managing wellness, social isolation and mental health. Anne has over 300 peer-reviewed journal articles as well as books on mental health, including the 6th edition of her prize winning and popular work, *A Sociology of Mental Health & Illness* (2021), and her latest book, *Living with Health Inequalities: Upstream-Downstream Connections* (2024).

Abbreviations

ADHD	Attention Deficit Hyperactivity Disorder
COPD	Chronic Obstructive Pulmonary Disease
HIV	Human Immunodeficiency Virus
ME/CFS	Myalgic encephalomyelitis/chronic fatigue syndrome
MS	Multiple Sclerosis
PCOS	Polycystic Ovarian Syndrome
PTSD	Post-Traumatic Stress Disorder
UK	United Kingdom
WHO	World Health Organisation

List of Figures

List of Tables

1

Introduction: Sick, lonely and left behind

The early twenty-first century has revealed a paradox of social connection: despite being more connected than ever before, many people feel more alone than in the past. Over time, perceptions about loneliness have shifted. During the nineteenth century, loneliness was viewed as an element of the human condition, as a state of ordinary distress, melancholy, sadness and angst. However, more recently, loneliness has been cast as a major social and health problem. Since the end of the twentieth century, there has been an exponential increase in attention to loneliness in research, politics, the media and public discourse. Loneliness is a pressing public policy issue globally (Goldman et al., 2024) with initiatives such as the World Health Organisation (WHO) Commission on Social Connection (WHO, 2025), national action plans in European countries (Velez & Euronews, 2023) and ministerial appointments in the UK (2018) and Japan (2021) to focus resources and combat the issue. The shift in loneliness from private and personal trouble to a social issue is also evident in the term "lonelygenic environments" (Feng & Astell-Burt, 2022) with loneliness attributed to a multiplicity of causal factors such as poor urban planning, remote work, social media use, austerity,

S. Lewis et al., *Unravelling the Layers of Chronic Illness and Loneliness*,
https://doi.org/10.1007/978-981-96-7909-6_1

poverty, racism, and xenophobia, declining collectivism and increasing individualism.

Loneliness is also viewed as a global public health problem. The significant costs and impacts of rising rates of loneliness have been likened to "a public health problem on the scale of smoking" (Lancet, 2023, p. 79). Policymakers, public health researchers, clinicians, and politicians have described loneliness as an "emerging epidemic" and the silent killer of our time (Cacioppo & Cacioppo, 2018; Sagan, 2023). In high-income countries, loneliness is reported to contribute to a range of social, economic and health problems from escalating mental illness, addiction and suicide rates, to the growing burden of chronic disease, "unhealthy" behaviours and social withdrawal, and mounting health and social care costs (Cacioppo & Cacioppo, 2014; Hawkley & Cacioppo, 2010; Holt-Lunstad et al., 2015; Wilson et al., 2007). In Australia, the economic costs of loneliness (primarily attributed to health care utilisation and adverse health behaviours among people who are lonely) are estimated at AUD$2.7 billion per year (Duncan et al., 2021). In the United States, estimates of economic impacts are US$154 billion (Office of the U.S. Surgeon General, 2023), while in the UK, the negative impact of severe loneliness has been estimated at £9,900 per year for each affected individual (Peytrignet et al., 2020).

People with chronic illnesses, such as diabetes, respiratory disorders, mental health conditions or chronic pain, are approximately twice as likely to experience chronic loneliness as those who do not experience chronic ill-health (Lim et al., 2023). Numerous studies have identified loneliness as one factor associated with conditions such as chronic pain (Allen et al., 2020; Consonni et al., 2021; Ong et al., 2021), type 2 diabetes (Christiansen et al., 2021), heart failure (Burström et al., 2012) and HIV (Leyva-Moral et al., 2019; Stroumpouki et al., 2020; Warren-Jeanpiere et al., 2014). People with chronic illnesses who are experiencing loneliness are reportedly more likely to call emergency services, be hospitalised, or visit their general practitioner, than those who are not lonely (Agarwal et al., 2019; Moseley et al., 2024; Parmar et al., 2022; Sirois & Owens, 2023). Loneliness is not restricted to those living with chronic illness. Their informal carers also experience the ill-effects of loneliness, with research showing increased visits to general practitioners, specialists and hospital among lonely carers compared to non-lonely carers (Majmadur et al., 2024). Yet, in clinical settings, the contextual aspects of loneliness are often missed, diagnosed as a mental illness (e.g. depression), or overlooked by clinicians (Kar-Lurkayastha, 2010). In the UK, general practitioners report an increasing number of patient visits due to loneliness but feel ill-equipped to provide appropriate support (Campaign to End Loneliness, 2013). Australian research indicates that health professionals place boundaries around what support they can provide to patients with chronic illnesses (e.g. managing symptoms to achieve clinical outcomes) but fail to recognise or act on references by their patients to loneliness (see Franklin et al., 2019). Such interactions result in patients feeling invisible, misunderstood or unsupported, while health professionals feeling frustrated by their inability to "fix" the problem.

Understanding Loneliness

Loneliness is most commonly defined as the subjective experience of dissatisfaction with the quality of one's social connections (De Jong Gierveld et al., 2006). Although the term loneliness is often used interchangeably with similar terms such as social isolation, these concepts are not the same. While social isolation refers primarily to a numerical lack of social connections, loneliness focuses attention to the negative experience of disconnectedness. Thus, Weiss (1973) viewed loneliness as a gnawing, chronic disease characterised by feelings of emptiness and abandonment. They drew a distinction between "emotional loneliness" stemming from the lack of an intimate relationship—typically a spouse, romantic partner or very close friend—and social loneliness as relational isolation stemming from the perceived and actual absence of a social network and consequential social ties (e.g. friends or familial connections) in one's life. From a psychological perspective, loneliness has been primarily defined as a subjective emotional state or adverse psychological response characterised by the painful feeling that arises when there is a felt difference between desired and actual social relationships (Russell et al., 1980). With the ascent of cognitive-behavioural therapy psychological perspectives shifted from early conceptions of loneliness as primarily emotional suffering to seeing loneliness as a potential precursor to mental illness (Seeman, 2022). Cognitive psychologists propose that loneliness is associated with neurobiological and behavioural factors which can lead to psychological reactions such as cognitive biases towards anticipating negative social interactions (the "self-fulfilling prophecy"), resulting in individuals avoiding social contact and thus reinforcing their experience of loneliness (Masi et al., 2011). Cacioppo and Hawkley (2009) propose that a recursive detrimental psychological impact of loneliness occurs because individuals are hyper-vigilant to social threat. As a result, people who are lonely can struggle to make accurate appraisals of social events, such that they (mis)interpret social events negatively and are "on the lookout" for negative social events so that they can avoid them to protect themselves from psychological pain (Cacioppo & Hawkley, 2009; Cacioppo et al., 2006).

Psychoanalytic approaches, which gained traction from the mid-twentieth century, also aligned loneliness with mental pathology. Loneliness was understood as linked to moods and feelings of alienation, anxiety and paranoia. Relationships with others in terms of care and nurturing came to be viewed as necessary for internal psychological well-being (VanBronkhorst et al., 2024). Loneliness was seen as rooted in biographical contexts of childhoods or in adults experiencing trauma or loss in the present. Through demonstrating the complex relationship between loneliness and early trauma, psychoanalytic research decoupled the construction of loneliness from its predominant conceptualisation as the outcome of a deficit of social connections (see Richards et al., 2013; Sagan, 2023). Psychoanalytic thinkers have also emphasised the importance of loneliness for personal growth and creativity, providing an alternative and more expansive understanding of loneliness (see Milton, 2018; Winnicott, 1958). Psychological perspectives have provided crucial insights into the internal mechanisms associated with loneliness, leading to personalised interventions targeting individual cognitions and behaviours. Over recent decades, psychologically based interventions have broadened to include social skills training and psychoeducation to ameliorate loneliness (Mann et al., 2017). However, viewing loneliness solely through a psychological lens risks privileging individual factors and pathologising loneliness, rather than addressing loneliness as inextricably linked to social environments.

Examining loneliness from a sociological perspective emphasises that it is a classical sociological problem—concerned with identifying, understanding and acting on the connections between seemingly "personal troubles" and the broader "public issues" that shape the personal (Wright Mills, 1959). Through the lens of the sociological imagination, loneliness can be viewed as a product of contemporary social life. This requires examination of the ideas that underpin our sense of self in society, the relationships that are valued, as well as the enduring and emerging societal (or structural) factors that can give rise to loneliness.

One of the first sociological theorists to identify societal influences on loneliness was Émile Durkheim. His study of suicide (1951 originally published in 1897) introduced concepts such as alienation and anomie, identifying how feeling cut off and adrift from society were important contributors to suicide. Berkman et al. (2000) argue that Durkheim's most important contribution was to understand "how social integration and cohesion influence mortality" and how "individual pathology was a function of social dynamics" (p. 844). The rootedness of loneliness in the social fabric was also highlighted by Simmel (1971 originally published in 1903) writing about city life at the turn of the twentieth century where: "one never feels as lonely and as deserted as in this metropolitan crush of persons" (p. 329). Simmel referred to a state of social isolation created by the heterogeneity of city life that replaced the uniformity and commonality of social bonds that bound people together under more traditional societal arrangements. The narrow, fleeting, and superficial interactions characteristic of city life produced circumstances in which people found it difficult to get to know one another, due to a lack of sufficient and meaningful contact during and as part of day-to-day activities (Simmel, 1908).

That loneliness is socially structured, rather than an individual condition, is the focus of work of sociologists such as Bauman (2012), Putnam (2015) and Franklin (2009). They identify a range of societal changes, including the rise of individualism, consumerism and reduced opportunities for social and civic participation, arguing that the resulting loss of social cohesion is a root cause for increasing rates of loneliness over time.

Putnam's (2015) study of social connectedness pointed to reductions in friendship and neighbour contact, conversational exchange in daily life, and familiarity with those around us. Similarly, the role of social networks in creating or ameliorating loneliness has also been explored. Social networks have the power to facilitate or restrict access to resources, emotional and instrumental support (Pescosolido, 2006). The interpersonal ties in social networks "provide sociability, support, information, a sense of belonging, norms and a social identity" (Wellman, 2000, p. 172).

Social networks vary across the life course and are subject to change through events, interpersonal dynamics and transitions in everyday lives (e.g. marriage, divorce, retirement, migration) which act as critical or trigger points that may increase the risk for loneliness. While social networks may be protective against loneliness, Cacioppo et al. (2009) claim they can also be a powerful mechanism for the social reproduction of loneliness. They pointed to social contagion, which they conceptualise as the spread of practices, behaviour, attitudes, and emotions through people's tendency to unconsciously adopt the behaviours and attitudes of others, as a mechanism in the spread of loneliness.

Individualising, Medicalising and Responsibilising Loneliness

With a focus on its harmful health consequences, the approaches to understanding and responding to loneliness have tended to perceive it as an individual pathology or personal deficit to be "treated", resulting in medicalisation and individualisation of loneliness (Victor et al., 2008). Instruments have been developed and psychometrically tested to measure loneliness. These measurements quantify loneliness within populations to help researchers and healthcare professionals better understand how loneliness affects health, identify risk factors, and evaluate the effectiveness of interventions aimed at reducing loneliness. These include the 20-item and revised 4-item UCLA Loneliness Scale (Russell et al., 1978, 1980), the De Jong Gierveld Loneliness Scale, an 11-item measure of both emotional and social loneliness (De Jong Gierveld &

van Tilburg, 1999), the 2014 Campaign to End Loneliness Measurement tool (Campaign to End Loneliness, n.d.) and other single-item measures (Ending Loneliness Together, 2021; Mund et al., 2023; Office for National Statistics, 2018). While tools such as these are designed for practical use (e.g. in service evaluations and by healthcare professionals), this method of understanding risks reinforcing loneliness as an intrinsically individual emotional state, linked to a lack of desired social connections (e.g. loss of, or separation from, loved ones).

These types of measures have limited capacity to capture the cultural and social variations in how loneliness is experienced and articulated. They have been critiqued for their tendency to homogenise the experience of loneliness, and inadequately capture or account for diverse loneliness experiences, trajectories and cultural contexts (Akhter-Khan & Au, 2020; Hymas et al., 2022). While some scales try to distinguish between different types of loneliness, many provide a single aggregate score that may oversimplify the complexity of the experience. In clinical settings, practitioners and primary care physicians are encouraged to screen patients for loneliness and to incorporate loneliness scales into chronic condition self-management care plans and consultations (Mullen et al., 2024). While greater attention to loneliness as a feature of the illness experience is important, when loneliness is understood and treated primarily as a psychological or medical issue of an individual atomised patient, without sufficient attention to socio-structural conditions that give rise to (or ameliorate loneliness), we risk framing it as primarily an issue of individual concern and responsibility.

Such framing is reflective of the neoliberal ideology entrenched in many modern societies across Australia, Europe and North America whereby individuals are expected to take chief responsibility for their economic, health and social outcomes, with reduced emphasis on the structural factors shaping these outcomes (Collyer et al., 2015). Neoliberal ideology (which posits that societies and economies should be arranged according to free market principles) has been associated with various austerity policies and retraction of government spending on public services, such as health care and social programs to encourage individual responsibility. Under neoliberalism, social disparities are seen as reflective of differences in hard work and deservedness, rather than differences in social and economic conditions (Collyer et al., 2015; Ostry et al., 2016). Neoliberal ideals of citizens who are autonomous, responsible, and independent are now part of the social, political and healthcare landscape, often under the guise of empowerment (Becker et al., 2021).

There is now extensive commentary on how neoliberal ideology contributes to loneliness. Becker et al. (2021) found that neoliberal ideology fuelled loneliness by reducing one's sense of connection, or solidarity, with others and increasing the sense that one is in competition with others. Peacock et al. (2014) argue that a neoliberal environment shapes discourses privileging the autonomous self to the extent that legitimacy of dependence upon others for care, support or sociability is "denied" and responsibility for life and life choices rests with individuals. Thus, Sagan (2023) argues that, rather than empowering individuals, there is a "moralist undertone" within neoliberal discourses that require individuals to manage their loneliness. Such discourses are also implicated in the stigma associated with loneliness (Barreto et al., 2022; Kerr & Stanley, 2021; Neves & Petersen, 2025). For Goffman (1963) stigma arises from specific attributes that are "deeply discrediting" (p. 3) which disqualify the individuals who bear these discrediting attributes, from complete social acceptance. For Barreto et al. (2022), loneliness-related stigma is "a constellation of beliefs that derogate and devalue those who feel lonely" (p. 2659). Such beliefs serve to ensure that individuals adhere to particular social standards of social connection to avoid the threat of social exclusion or marginalisation (see also Phelan et al., 2008). The shame and stigma surrounding loneliness, in this context, means that individuals who are lonely are deemed to have failed to self-manage their sociability, and as Neves and Petersen (2025) point out in the case of older people, the label of loneliness reinforces stereotypes and discrimination. In a context where "sociability, productivity and young healthy bodies" are valued, identity management such as concealment of loneliness occurs in order "to avoid a sense of personal failure or demise" (Neves & Petersen, 2025, pp. 12–13).

Many people with chronic illnesses may already be marginalised and excluded from mainstream society due to illnesses that are deemed to breach social norms (e.g. many mental illnesses) or that are attributed to so-called lifestyle factors (e.g. chronic obstructive pulmonary disease, type 2 diabetes) (Dolezal, 2022); thus, the stigma and shame associated with being *both* lonely and sick can act as a double burden to manage. Additionally, the poor health and functional limitations that come with chronic illness, such as fatigue or pain, coupled with the invisibility, shame and/or stigma of living with illness, can result in loneliness, seriously diminishing the quality of a person's relationships, the frequency of their social contact with others, and their ability or desire to participate in their social worlds (De Jong Gierveld et al., 2006).

Coinciding with the increasing trend towards framing loneliness as an individual concern and responsibility, there has been a trend over the past twenty years for loneliness to be framed in public discourse as a medical problem (Sagan, 2023).This medicalisation of loneliness is evident in, for example, portrayals of loneliness in the mass media as pandemic, health crisis or moral panic; the focus in scientific research (e.g. neuroscience research on protein factors linked to loneliness) (Gong et al., 2025) and the search for solutions such as "the loneliness pill" (Carney, 2020). Within medicine, approaches to reducing loneliness include individual counselling, new mobile and digital health technologies, and pharmaceutical treatments; all of which aim to address loneliness by fixing the lonely individual, primarily through providing them with the tools to become more socially connected (Hawkley & Cacioppo, 2010).

One effect of the discourse focused on fixing individuals, is that we are told we can think, feel, or act our way out of being lonely; and this perspective is evident across a burgeoning popular literature on the topic. There is now a "loneliness economy" comprising self-help books, workshops and podcasts. The focus is firmly on personal experiences and the individual taking personal responsibility for their loneliness through changing thoughts or behaviours. A perusal of just about any bookshop will offer numerous publications, ranging from scholarly intervention studies by researcher clinicians advocating "self-help" approaches to combatting loneliness, to self-help books written sometimes by experts and sometimes by lay people (often touting "solutions" or even a "cure" for loneliness), and books written by experts for clinicians/counsellors to give them strategies for helping their patients/clients. While on the surface this discourse appears to be empowering, the lack of attention to social context places responsibility onto individuals to undertake the steps needed to ameliorate their loneliness. Other approaches emphasising the social aspects of loneliness by enhancing connection, engagement with social activities, community assets, and social identification with neighbourhood (see, e.g. Band & Rogers, 2024; Fong et al., 2021; Noone & Yang, 2022) receive less attention in the public conceptualisation of loneliness.

Chronic Condition Care and Loneliness

The increased prevalence and burden of chronic conditions poses challenges for both individuals and healthcare systems. The biomedical approach focuses on the diagnosis and treatment of disease in clinical settings, relying on surgical, genetic, pharmaceutical interventions, and individual behaviour changes. There is now acknowledgement in policies of the shortcomings of this approach in providing good care to people with chronic conditions (Australian Health Ministers' Advisory Council, 2017; National Health Priority Action Council, 2006; Willcox, 2014), with emphasis on the importance of tailoring chronic condition support to the needs of people who are socially marginalised and particular attention on the negative impacts of socio-economic disadvantage (Willcox, 2014). Despite this, policies such as the Australian Health Minister's Advisory Council's (2017) *National Strategic Framework for Chronic Conditions* lack specific guidance on how to practically address the underlying social impacts of living with chronic conditions, such as loneliness, social isolation and lack of social support. There is no mention of loneliness in this Framework.

An enduring trope across chronic disease national strategies, in Australia and many other countries, has been the emphasis on self-management strategies to encourage individuals to take more personal responsibility for their conditions (Australian Health Minister's Advisory Council, 2017). Chronic condition self-management is predicated on active patient involvement in managing symptoms, adopting healthy lifestyles, and seeking medical support (Franklin et al., 2019). Successful self-management requires individual attributes such as being future-oriented, proactive and independent. When loneliness is addressed from within such a framework, it becomes an extension of being the "responsible self-manager". Yet, viewing loneliness as socially situated and experienced, demands a different approach.

A range of programs and initiatives across healthcare and community settings have sought to respond to loneliness as part of chronic condition care and support. Social prescribing, the harnessing of assets and resources in the community sector to encourage social connectivity for those experiencing loneliness (Morse et al., 2022), is increasingly being adopted by practitioners to address gaps in self-management support (Gottlieb et al., 2018). It draws on the possibilities of social engagement as a potent mechanism for connecting people into the community (Lester et al., 2012). Although a focus on social connection is positive, a key critique of social prescribing is that, like chronic condition self-management, it assumes a high degree of patient agency and that people have equal opportunity to mobilise the resources they need to be more socially engaged. It also increases health professionals' responsibility to attend to social issues.

Similarly, digital health technologies (e.g. mHealth and web-based support groups) are sometimes seen to be aligned with person-centred approaches to health care and transformative in their potential to increase social connectivity and/or remedy loneliness for patients, as well as reduce healthcare costs. Digital scholars have examined the complex ways in which technologies may enhance, transform, but also disrupt and hinder social connection in different illness contexts (Allen et al., 2019). Yet, in our hyper-connected digital world, disentangling the complexities of digital technologies, spaces and connections—including how they help, hinder or otherwise mediate experiences of loneliness for those with chronic illness is challenging. The development and use of various digital "solutions" to loneliness outpaces the accumulation of evidence to support their effectiveness (Neves et al., 2024).

Community-based programs and interventions have sought to bridge health and community care and support. For example, interventions that utilise the power of peer support (Hossain et al., 2021; Kingod et al., 2017; Thompson et al., 2022) and social networks (Ellis et al., 2020;

Welch et al., 2021), recognise the importance of cultivating meaningful social activities and relationships in ameliorating loneliness. Health condition-specific cafes offer informal, community-based spaces where those affected by chronic health conditions and families and carers can connect while accessing professional support (Greenwood et al., 2017; Takechi et al., 2018). Nature-based programs have also been designed to facilitate connection with the natural world and non-human beings (Litt et al., 2024; Sachs et al., 2024), recognising the importance of non-human relationships and connections in alleviating loneliness.

These approaches are promising because they seek to embed responses to loneliness within people's daily lives, local environments and wider social contexts by recognising the importance of focusing on what is meaningful to individuals and communities. However, evidence of their effectiveness, especially over the longer term, is mixed. Common challenges persist across these approaches including accommodating illness fluctuations, finding accessible venues and securing sustainable funding. Additionally, most interventions and programs still primarily focus on later life, meaning that there is a lack of initiatives to tackle loneliness for people with chronic illnesses across the life course. Despite growing interest in the topic of loneliness, there remains a need for greater attention to how loneliness is implicated in the chronic illness experience, including the social factors that contribute to loneliness and ways to effectively respond to it as a social problem.

This Book

The relationship between chronic illness and loneliness is complex and bi-directional but still not well understood, especially from a social perspective. What is less explored is the complex mix of personal, interpersonal and social factors that contribute to people with chronic illnesses being lonely (Neves & Petersen, 2025; Sagan, 2023). These factors include the interwoven effects of immobility, psychological distress, loss of self, stigmatisation and institutional discrimination, as well as the structuring of health care which places a high value on individual autonomy and independence (Barlow et al., 2015). The relationship between loneliness and chronic illness is also recursive—with many people stuck in a downward spiral of worsening health and increased loneliness (Malli et al., 2022). For many, chronic illness and loneliness interact producing worsening health and social outcomes and those with less capacity to change their circumstances, with fewer social and economic resources to mobilise, are more vulnerable. Yet despite increased recognition that people with chronic illnesses are disproportionally affected by loneliness and its adverse consequences, there remains little research, especially from a social perspective, on how people with chronic illnesses (and those who care and support them) experience loneliness in their everyday lives and what it means to them. Loneliness is replete with social meanings; it is constructed, interpreted and experienced variously by multiple social actors (people with different types of chronic illnesses, family members, friends, health professionals, and others providing care and support) and involves personal, interpersonal, temporal, and social dimensions.

In this book, we draw on empirical data to conceptualise loneliness as relationally experienced, shaped by illness trajectories, social stigma, social expectations and values, life histories, place, digital worlds, expectations for care and social support. In conceptualising loneliness as a social issue, emphasising its relational and societal nature (see also Rogers & Pilgrim, 2023) we frame loneliness as emerging through the dynamic interaction between person, experience, and social context (Valenzuela-Garcia et al., 2021). A relational approach attends to human relationships and the networks of relationships and interactions between multiple human and non-human actors. It acknowledges how experiences of loneliness shape and are shaped by individual biography, life history, geography and social positioning (Franklin & Tranter, 2021; Neves et al., 2019).

This book draws on fieldwork from a large qualitative study conducted between 2020 and 2025 as part of an Australian Research Council Discovery Grant titled "Sick, lonely and left behind: A sociological study of loneliness". This multi-stage study sought to explore the perspectives of people with chronic illnesses who were experiencing loneliness, the meanings they gave to these experiences, and propose strategies important in alleviating loneliness among this group. We also interviewed informal carers and health and community care professionals who shared their insights about their roles and experiences in providing care and support to those with chronic illnesses and experiencing loneliness.

We interviewed 40 people (28 women, 11 men, and one non-binary person) with a diverse range of chronic physical and mental health conditions and who self-identified as lonely or disconnected. A strength of our longitudinal approach was interviewing participants up to three times over a 12-month period, allowing us to identify and reflect on changes in participants' experiences over time. Interviews were conducted in a location chosen by the participant or via videoconferencing. Some participants also participated in walking interviews, photo elicitation or completed daily diaries documenting their experiences. Participants ranged in age between 19 and 83 years, resided in a range of geographic locations (e.g. urban, regional or rural), were diverse in socio-demographic characteristics, such as relationship status, ethnicity, socio-economic status, and time since diagnosis of their condition. Most participants were living with more than one chronic condition. A table of participant characteristics is included in Table 1 in the Appendix. Interviews explored experiences of health, illness, health care, loneliness, beliefs about loneliness, strategies for managing feelings of loneliness, social networks and experiences of social relationships and supports, as well as places and spaces that were meaningful for their experience of chronic illness, loneliness, and feeling socially connected.

We also interviewed 27 family members and other informal carers who were providing support and care for a person living with a chronic illness (25 females and 2 men, ranging in age from 24 to 74 years). Participants were caring for a range of family members including their mother, father, son, daughter, sister, grandmother, wife, husband or friend living with a diversity of chronic health conditions. See Table 2 (in Appendix) for carer participant characteristics. Interviews were conducted either in-person, over the phone or via videoconferencing. These interviews explored carers' perspectives on loneliness, the strategies they used to address the loneliness of the person they were caring for, and the impacts of loneliness on the relationship between carers and people living with chronic illness.

Interviews were conducted with 23 health and community care professionals. Participants included medical professionals, nurses, allied health professionals and community workers working in the public, private and not-for-profit sectors in a mix of metropolitan, regional, rural or remote areas in Australia (see Table 3 in Appendix for participant characteristics). Interviews were conducted via phone or videoconferencing. These participants provided health care and support for people living with a diverse range of chronic physical and mental health conditions and/or intellectual, physical, and developmental disability. Interviews explored professionals' experiences providing support for people feeling lonely or isolated, how they recognised loneliness and isolation in clients, which tools they drew on to talk to clients about their loneliness, and the resources and information they found helpful to support such conversations.

The Contents of the Book

In drawing on the perspectives of those with lived experience of chronic illness and loneliness, their carers and health professionals, we have chosen to use the term chronic illness as an umbrella term to describe an illness or disease (such as multiple sclerosis, diabetes, mental health condition, rheumatoid arthritis) that lasts for a long period (typically more than 6 months), that usually requires ongoing medical management and has an impact on the person's daily life and functioning. While in the literature chronic illness is often used interchangeably with other terms like chronic health condition and long-term health condition, the term chronic illness places an emphasis on the lived experience of illness and foregrounds lived experiences and subjective meanings. It is also the term used in many patient and consumer advocacy contexts. Throughout the book, we use quotes from participants to illuminate our learnings from them. The names used are pseudonyms, details that may be identifying have been removed and only overview data are provided (such as age range, rather than specific age).

Chapters Two, Three and Four focus on various dimensions of loneliness as experienced by participants with chronic illnesses. In Chapter Two, we discuss how participants in our research described and gave meaning to the experience of chronic conditions and loneliness. Three broad, sometimes overlapping, themes illustrate their loneliness—personally, as feeling insignificant, damaged, or "broken"; socially, as irrelevant to others; and societally, as alienated from participation in society. Chapter Three explores chronicity and loneliness through a temporal lens illustrating how assumptions of linear and sequential life progression stand in tension with the messiness of the lived experience of chronic conditions. We show how experiences of illness shift one's sense of belonging in the world (and in the imagined future life course) with loneliness occurring through a sense of being left behind in the present, experienced through the lens of their past and their uncertainty about the future. In Chapter Four, we examine the complexities of social relationships in experiences of loneliness and social support. We unpack how issues of authenticity, interdependency and reciprocity are related to forming and maintaining meaningful social bonds as participants describe changing relationships, the work required to manage relationships, the support they need and the importance of connections beyond humans, including relationships with other animals.

Chapters Five, Six and Seven extend the discussion of dimensions of loneliness, to examine how people with chronic conditions manage loneliness. Chapter Five discusses the broad strategies revealed by study participants that help alleviate loneliness. We argue that strategies to overcome loneliness are also part of the identity work that individuals must engage in to carefully craft their presentation of self in social situations. This occurs not only because of the expectations held by family and friends, but also due to the expectations they hold for themselves. In Chapter Six, we turn our attention to how participants valued and engaged with digital technologies and spaces, capturing how digital spaces enhance as well as hinder connectedness, and the complexities and underlying tensions associated with digital connectivity and chronic illness. In Chapter Seven, we examine the relevance of place and neighbourhood in the experience of loneliness. Data from our interviews is organised around the types of places important to participants—the home and neighbourhood, places of purpose and recognition (these include places of work and health facilities), and public places outside of home and work where people can seek meaning in nature, where they can have fleeting, incidental interactions, or where they can choose to be sociable.

In Chapters Eight and Nine, we draw on interviews with informal carers and health and community care professionals respectively to examine care relationships. In Chapter Eight we present findings from interviews with informal carers where we examined the work of family members and other informal carers. We show how loneliness is implicated in the experience of being a carer, the expectations and responses which contribute to a loss of self outside of their carer identity, their sense of responsibility to care well and a feeling of invisibility in social interactions. In Chapter Nine, we focus on the professional workforce, drawing on data from interviews with health and community care professionals. The chapter examines how health professionals identify and respond to experiences of loneliness for people living with chronic conditions. We show that while professionals do care about the dynamic interplay between loneliness and living with a long-term condition, many are constrained in how they can attend to loneliness in their interactions with people living with chronic conditions.

In Chapter Ten, we conclude by synthesising the key arguments made throughout the book and examine how models of policy and practice might be changed to better incorporate the care and support needs of people with chronic conditions who experience loneliness. We argue there is an imperative for community strategies to address loneliness and the need to take a relational approach to loneliness that attends to the broader systemic forces driving loneliness among those with chronic conditions.

References

Akhter-Khan, S. C., & Au, R. (2020). Why loneliness interventions are unsuccessful: A call for precision health. *Advances in Geriatric Medicine and Research, 2*(3), e200016. https://doi.org/10.20900/agmr20200016

Allen, C., Vassilev, I., Kennedy, A., & Rogers, A. (2019). The work and relatedness of ties mediated online in supporting long-term condition self-management. *Sociology of Health & Illness, 42*(3), 579–595. https://doi.org/10.1111/1467-9566.13042

Allen, S. F., Gilbody, S., Atkin, K., & van der Feltz-Cornelis, C. (2020). The associations between loneliness, social exclusion and pain in the general population: A N=502,528 cross-sectional UK Biobank study. *Journal of Psychiatric Research, 130*, 68–74.

Agarwal, G., Lee, J., McLeod, B., Mahmuda, S., Howard, M., Cockrell, K., & Angeles, R. (2019). Social factors in frequent callers: A description of isolation, poverty and quality of life in those calling emergency medical services frequently. *BMC Public Health, 19*, 1–8.

Australian Health Ministers' Advisory Council. (2017). *National Strategic Framework for Chronic Conditions*. Australian Government. Canberra. https://www.health.gov.au/resources/publications/national-strategic-framework-for-chronic-conditions?language=en

Band, R., & Rogers, A. (2024). Understanding the meaning of loneliness and social engagement for the workings of a social network intervention connecting people to resources and valued activities. *Health Expectations, 27*(6), Article e70111. https://doi.org/10.1111/hex.70111

Barreto, M., van Breen, J., Victor, C., Hammond, C., Eccles, A., Richins, M. T., & Qualter, P. (2022). Exploring the nature and variation of the stigma associated with loneliness. *Journal of Social and Personal Relationships, 39*(9), 2658–2679. https://doi.org/10.1177/02654075221087190

Barlow, M. A., Liu, S. Y., & Wrosch, C. (2015). Chronic illness and loneliness in older adulthood: The role of self-protective control strategies. *Health Psychology, 34*(8), 870–879.

Bauman, Z. (2012). *Liquid Modernity*. Polity Press, Cambridge (original date of publication 2000).

Becker, J. C., Hartwich, L., & Haslam, S. A. (2021). Neoliberalism can reduce well-being by promoting a sense of social disconnection, competition, and loneliness. *British Journal of Social Psychology, 60*(3), 947–965.

Berkman, L., Glass, T., Brissette, I., & Seeman, T. (2000). From social integration to health: Durkheim in the new millennium. *Social Science and Medicine, 51*, 843–857.

Burström, M., Brännström, M., Boman, K., & Strandberg, G. (2012). Life experiences of security and insecurity among women with chronic heart failure. *Journal of Advanced Nursing, 68*(4), 816–825. https://doi.org/10.1111/j.1365-2648.2011.05782.x

Cacioppo, J. T., & Cacioppo, S. (2014). Social relationships and health: The toxic effects of perceived social isolation. *Social and Personality Psychology Compass, 8*(2), 58–72. https://doi.org/10.1111/spc3.12087

Cacioppo, J. T., & Cacioppo, S. (2018). The growing problem of loneliness. *Lancet, 391*(10119), 426.

Cacioppo, J. T., Fowler, J. H., & Christiakis, N. A. (2009). Alone in the crowd: The structure and spread of loneliness in a large social network. *Journal of Personality and Social Psychology, 97*(6), 977–999.

Cacioppo, J. T., & Hawkley, L. (2009). Perceived social isolation and cognition. *Trends in Cognitive Sciences, 13*(10), 447–454. https://doi.org/10.1016/j.tics.2009.06.005

Cacioppo, J. T., Hawkley, L. C., Ernst, J. M., Burleson, M., Berntson, G. G., Nouriani, B., & Spiegel, D. (2006). Loneliness within a nomological net: An evolutionary perspective. *Journal of Research in Personality, 40*(6), 1054–1085.

Campaign to End Loneliness. (2013). *Family doctors ill-equipped for loneliness epidemic* [Press release]. https://www.campaigntoendloneliness.org/wp-content/uploads/downloads/2013/11/FINAL-GP-Polling-PR-15.11.13.pdf

Campaign to End Loneliness (n.d.). *Measuring your impact on loneliness in later life.* https://www.campaigntoendloneliness.org/wp-content/uploads/Loneliness-Measurement-Guidance1.pdf

Carney, A., (2020). *Can loneliness be cured with a pill? Scientists are now asking the question.* The Guardian. Retrieved 29 January, 2025 from https://www.theguardian.com/lifeandstyle/2020/aug/06/loneliness-cure-pill-research-scientists

Christiansen, J., Lund, R., Qualter, P., Andersen, C., Pedersen, S. S., & Lasgaard, M. (2021). Loneliness, social isolation, and chronic disease outcomes. *Annals of Behavioral Medicine, 55*(3), 203–215.

Collyer, F. M., Willis, K. F., Franklin, M., Harley, K., & Short, S. D. (2015). Healthcare choice: Bourdieu's capital, habitus and field. *Contemporary Sociology, 63*(5), 685–699.

Consonni, M., Telesca, A., Grazzi, L., Cazzato, D., & Lauria, G. (2021). Life with chronic pain during COVID-19 lockdown: The case of patients with small fibre neuropathy and chronic migraine. *Neurological Sciences, 42*(2), 389–397.

De Jong Gierveld, J., & van Tilburg, T. G. (1999). *Manual of the loneliness scale*. Methoden en technieken. https://doi.org/10.17605/osf.io/u6gck

De Jong Gierveld, J., van Tilburg, T. G., & Dykstra, P. A. (2006). Loneliness and social isolation. In D. Perlman & A. Vangelisti (Eds.), *The Cambridge handbook of personal relationships* (pp. 485–500). Cambridge University Press.

Dolezal, L. (2022). Shame anxiety, stigma and clinical encounters. *Journal of Evaluation in Clinical Practice, 28*, 854–860.

Duncan, A., Kiely, D., Mavisakalyan, A., Peters, A., Seymour, R., Twomey, C., & Vu, L. (2021). *Stronger together: Loneliness and social connectedness in Australia. Bankwest Curtin Economics Centre Focus on the State Series, #8, November 2021.* https://bcec.edu.au/publications/stronger-together-loneliness-and-social-connectedness-in-australia/

Durkheim, E. (1951). *Suicide: A study in sociology.*, 2nd edition. Routledge. https://doi.org/10.4324/9780203994320

Ellis, J., Band, R., Kinsella, K., Cheetham-Blake, T., James, E., Ewings, S., & Rogers, A. (2020). Optimising and profiling pre-implementation contexts to create and implement a public health network intervention for tackling loneliness. *Implementation Science*. https://doi.org/10.1186/s13012-020-00997-x

Ending Loneliness Together (2021). *A guide to evaluating loneliness outcomes for community organisations.* https://endingloneliness.com.au/wp-content/uploads/2021/08/A-Guide-to-Measuring-Loneliness-for-Community-Organisations_Ending-Loneliness-Together.pdf

Feng, X., & Astell-Burt, T. (2022). Lonelygenic environments: A call for research on multilevel determinants of loneliness. *The Lancet. Planetary Health, 6*(12), e933–e934.

Franklin, A. S. (2009). On loneliness. *Geografiska Annaler: Series b, Human Geography, 91*(4), 343–354. https://doi.org/10.1111/j.1468-0467.2009.00326.x

Franklin, M., Lewis, S., Willis, K., Rogers, A., Venville, A., & Smith, L. (2019). Goals for living with a chronic condition: The relevance of temporalities, dispositions, and resources. *Social Science & Medicine, 233*, 13–20.

Franklin, A., & Tranter, B. (2021). Loneliness and the cultural, spatial, temporal and generational bases of belonging. *Australian Journal of*

Psychology, *73*(6), 1–13. http://dx.doi.org/10.1080/00049530.2020.1837007

Fong, P., Cruwys, T., Robinson, S. L., Haslam, S. A., Haslam, C., Mance, P. L., & Fisher, C. L. (2021). Evidence that loneliness can be reduced by a whole-of-community intervention to increase neighbourhood identification. *Soc Science & Medicine, 277*, Article 113909. https://doi.org/10.1016/j.socscimed.2021.113909

Goffman, E. (1963). *Stigma: Notes on the management of spoiled identity.* Penguin Books.

Goldman, N., Khanna, D., El Asmar, M. L., Qualter, P., & El-Osta, A. (2024). Addressing loneliness and social isolation in 52 countries: A scoping review of national policies. *BMC Public Health.* https://doi.org/10.1186/s12889-024-18370-8

Gong, J., Preminger, Z., Steptoe, A., & Fancourt, D. (2025). Protein signatures associated with loneliness and social isolation: Plasma proteome analyses in the English Longitudinal Study of Ageing, with causal evidence from Mendelian randomization. *Brain, Behavior, and Immunity, 124*, 85–94.

Gottlieb, L., Cottrell, E. K., Park, B., Clark, K. D., Gold, R., & Fichtenberg, C. (2018). Advancing social prescribing with implementation science. *Journal of the American Board of Family Medicine, 31*(3), 315–321. https://doi.org/10.3122/jabfm.2018.03.170249

Greenwood, N., Smith, R., Akhtar, F., & Richardson, A. (2017). A qualitative study of carers' experiences of dementia cafes: A place to feel supported and be yourself. *BMC Geriatrics, 17*(1), 164. https://doi.org/10.1186/s12877-017-0559-4

Haslam, S. A., McMahon, C., Cruwys, T., Haslam, C., Jetten, J., & Steffens, N. K. (2018). Social cure, what social cure? The propensity to underestimate the importance of social factors for health. *Social Science & Medicine, 198*, 14–21.

Hawkley, L. C., & Cacioppo, J. T. (2010). Loneliness matters: A theoretical and empirical review of consequences and mechanisms. *Annals of Behavioral Medicine, 40*(2), 218–227. https://doi.org/10.1007/s12160-010-9210-8

Holt-Lunstad, J., Smith, T. B., Baker, M., Harris, T., & Stephenson, D. (2015). Loneliness and social isolation as risk factors for mortality: A meta-analytic review. *Perspectives on Psychological Science, 10*(2), 227–237. https://doi.org/10.1177/1745691614568352

Hossain, S. N., Jaglal, S. B., Shepherd, J., Perrier, L., Tomasone, J. R., Sweet, S. N., & Munce, S. E. (2021). Web-based peer support interventions for adults living with chronic conditions: Scoping review. *JMIR Rehabilitation and Assistive Technologies, 8*(2), Article e14321.

Hughes, S., Lewis, S., Willis, K., Rogers, A., Wyke, S., & Smith, L. (2020). Goal setting in group programmes for long-term condition self-management support: Experiences of patients and healthcare professionals. *Psychology & Health, 35*(1), 70–86.

Hymas, R., Badcock, J. C., & Milne, E. (2022). Loneliness in autism and its association with anxiety and depression: A systematic review with meta-analyses. *Review Journal of Autism and Developmental Disorders, 11*, 121–156. https://doi.org/10.1007/s40489-022-00330-w

Kar-Purkayastha, I. (2010). An epidemic of loneliness. *Lancet, 376*(9758), 2114–2115. https://doi.org/10.1016/S0140-6736(10)62190-3

Kerr, N. A., & Stanley, T. B. (2021). Revisiting the social stigma of loneliness. *Personality and Individual Differences, 171*(3), 110482.

Kingod, N., Cleal, B., Wahlberg, A., & Husted, G. R. (2017). Online peer-to-peer communities in the daily lives of people with chronic illness: A qualitative systematic review. *Qualitative Health Research, 27*(1), 89–99.

Leyva-Moral, J. M., Martínez-Batlle, F., Vázquez-Naveira, M., Hernández-Fernández, J., & Villar-Salgueiro, M. (2019). The experience of growing old while living with HIV in Spain: A phenomenological study. *Journal of the Association of Nurses in AIDS Care, 30*(1), 111–118. https://doi.org/10.1097/JNC.0000000000000032

Lancet, T. (2023). Loneliness as a health issue. *The Lancet Editorial, 402*(10396), 79.

Lester, H., Mead, N., Graham, C. C., Gask, L., & Reilly, S. (2012). An exploration of the value and mechanisms of befriending for older adults in England. *Ageing & Society, 32*(2), 307–328.

Lim, M. H., Qualter, P., Ding, D., Holt-Lunstad, J., Mikton, C., & Smith, B. J. (2023). Advancing loneliness and social isolation as global health challenges: Taking three priority actions. *Public Health Research & Practice, 33*(3), e3332320. https://doi.org/10.17061/phrp3332320

Litt, J. S., Coll-Planas, L., Sachs, A. L., Rochau, U., Jansson, A., Dostálová, V., & Pitkälä, K. H. (2024). Nature-based social interventions for people experiencing loneliness: The rationale and overview of the RECETAS project. *Cities & Health, 8*(3), 418–431. https://doi.org/10.1080/23748834.2023.2300207

Majmadur, I. K., Mihalopoulos, C., Abimanyi-Ochom, J., Mohebbi, M., & Engel, L. (2024). The association between loneliness with health service use and quality of life among informal carers in Australia. *Social Science &*

Medicine, 348, Article 116821. https://doi.org/10.1016/j.socscimed.2024.116821
Malli, M. A., Ryan, S., Maddison, J., & Kharicha, K. (2022). Experiences and meaning of loneliness beyond age and group identity. *Sociology and Health & Illness, 45*(1), 70–89.
Mann, F., Bone, J. K., Lloyd-Evans, B., Frerichs, J., Pinfold, V., Ma, R., & Johnson, S. (2017). A life less lonely: The state of the art in interventions to reduce loneliness in people with mental health problems. *Social Psychiatry and Psychiatric Epidemiology, 52*, 627–638. https://doi.org/10.1007/s00127-017-1392-y
Masi, C. M., Chen, H. Y., Hawkley, L. C., & Cacioppo, J. T. (2011). A meta-analysis of interventions to reduce loneliness. *Personality and Social Psychology Review, 15*, 219–266.
Milton, J. (2018). From the Melanie Klein archive: Klein's further thoughts on loneliness. *The International Journal of Psychoanalysis, 99*(4), 929–946.
Morse, D. F., Sandhu, S., Mulligan, K., Tierney, S., Polley, M., Chiva Giurca, B., & Slade, S. (2022). Global developments in social prescribing. *BMJ Global Health*, 7(5), e008524. https://doi.org/10.1136/bmjgh-2022-008524
Moseley, L., Scott, J., Fidler, G., Agarwal, G., Clarke, C., Hammond-Williams, J., & Collins, T. (2024). 'If it was easy somebody would have fixed it': An exploration of loneliness and social isolation amongst people who frequently call ambulance services. *Health Expectations, 27*(4), Article e14167.
Mullen, R. A., Tong, S. T., Lum, H. D., Stephens, K. A., & Krist, A. H. (2024). The role of primary care in the social isolation and loneliness epidemic. *The Annals of Family Medicine, 22*(3), 244–246.
Mund, M., Maes, M., Drewke, P. M., Gutzeit, A., Jaki, I., & Qualter, P. (2023). Would the real loneliness please stand up? The validity of loneliness scores and the reliability of single-item scores. *Assessment, 30*(4), 1226–1248.
National Health Priority Action Council (NHPAC) (2006), *National Chronic Disease Strategy*, Australian Government Department of Health and Ageing, Canberra. https://www.health.gov.au/sites/default/files/documents/2019/09/national-strategic-framework-for-chronic-conditions.pdf
Neves, B. B., Sanders, A., & Kokanović, R. (2019). "It's the worst bloody feeling in the world": Experiences of loneliness and social isolation among older people living in care homes. *Journal of Aging Studies, 49*, 74–84.
Neves, B. B., Sanders, A., Warren, N., & Ko, P. C. (2024). Loneliness in later life as existential inequality. *Sociology, 58*, 659.
Neves, B. B., & Petersen, A. (2025). The social stigma of loneliness: A sociological approach to understanding the experiences of older people.

The Sociological Review. 73(2), 362-383. https://doi.org/10.1177/003802612312121
Noone, C., & Yang, K. (2022). Community-based responses to loneliness in older people: A systematic review of qualitative studies. *Health & Social Care in the Community, 30*, e859–e873. https://doi.org/10.1111/hsc.13682
Office for National Statistics (2018). *Measuring loneliness: Guidance for use of the national indicators on surveys.* https://www.ons.gov.uk/peoplepopulationandcommunity/wellbeing/methodologies/measuringlonelinessguidanceforuseofthenationalindicatorsonsurveys
Office of the U.S. Surgeon General (2023). *Our epidemic of loneliness and isolation. The U.S. Surgeon General's Advisory on the healing effects of social connection and community.* U.S. Department of Health and Human Services. https://www.hhs.gov/sites/default/files/surgeon-general-social-connection-advisory.pdf
Ong, A. D., Goktas, S., & Reid, M. C. (2021). More than hurt feelings: The wear and tear of day-to-day discrimination in adults with chronic pain. *Pain Medicine, 22*(12), 2925–2930.
Ostry, J. D., Loungani, P., & Furceri, D. (2016). Neoliberalism: Oversold? Instead of delivering growth, some neoliberal policies have increased inequality, in turn jeopardizing durable expansion. *Finance & Development, 53*(2), 38–42.
Parmar, M., Ma, R., Attygalle, S., Mueller, C., Stubbs, B., Stewart, R., & Perera, G. (2022). Associations between loneliness and acute hospitalisation outcomes among patients receiving mental healthcare in South London: A retrospective cohort study. *Social Psychiatry and Psychiatric Epidemiology, 57*(2), 397–410. https://doi.org/10.1007/s00127-021-02079-9
Peacock, M., Bissell, P., & Owen, J. (2014). Dependency denied: Health inequalities in the neo-liberal era. *Social Science and Medicine, 118*, 173–180.
Pescosolido, B. A. (2006). Of pride and prejudice: The role of sociology and social networks in integrating the health sciences. *Journal of Health and Social Behavior, 47*(3), 189–208. https://doi.org/10.1177/002214650604700301
Peytrignet, S., Garforth-Bles, S., & Keohane, K. (2020). *Loneliness monetisation report.* Simetrica. HM Government, United Kingdom. https://www.gov.uk/government/publications/loneliness-monetisation-report
Phelan, J. C., Link, B. G., & Dovidio, J. F. (2008). Stigma and prejudice: One animal or two? *Social Science & Medicine, 67*(3), 358–367.

Putnam, R. D. (2015). Bowling alone: America's declining social capital. In *The city reader* (pp. 188–196). Routledge
Richards, A. K., Spira, L., & Lynch, A. (Eds). (2013). The clinical dimensions of loneliness. In *Encounters with loneliness: Only the lonely* (2nd ed., pp. 51–65). International Psychoanalytic Books.
Rogers, A., & Pilgrim, D. (2023). *Living with health inequalities: Upstream-downstream connections.* Routledge.
Russell, D., Peplau, L. A., & Ferguson, M. L. (1978). Developing a measure of loneliness. *Journal of Personality Assessment, 42*(3), 290–294. https://doi.org/10.1207/s15327752jpa4203_11
Russell, D., Peplau, L. A., & Cutrona, C. E. (1980). The revised UCLA loneliness scale: Concurrent and discriminant validity evidence. *Journal of Personality and Social Psychology, 39*(3), 472–480. https://doi.org/10.1037/0022-3514.39.3.472
Sachs, A. L., Kolster, A., Wrigley, J., Papon, V., Opacin, N., Hill, N., & Litt, J. (2024). Connecting through nature: A systematic review of the effectiveness of nature-based social prescribing practices to combat loneliness. *Landscape and Urban Planning, 248*, Article 105071.
Sagan, O. (2023). Organised loneliness and its discontents. *Diversity & Inclusion Research, 1*(1), Article e12008. https://doi.org/10.1002/dvr2.12008
Seeman, A. (2022). The psychological structure of loneliness. *International Journal of Environmental Research and Public Health, 19*(3), 1061. https://doi.org/10.3390/ijerph19031061
Simmel, G. (1971). The metropolis and mental Life, trans. Edward S. Shils. In G. Simmel (Ed.), *On Individuality and Social Forms*, edited with an Introduction by Donald. N. Levine, (pp. 324–339). Chicago University Press
Simmel, G. (1908). *The sociology of Georg Simmel* (K. Wolff, Trans.). Free Press.
Sirois, F. M., & Owens, J. (2023). A meta-analysis of loneliness and use of primary health care. *Health Psychology Review, 17*(2), 193–210.
Stroumpouki, T., Perrett, S., Kasdovasilis, P., Papatheodorou, P., Paparizos, V., & Stavropoulou, A. (2020). A journey towards acceptance: The process of adapting to life with HIV in Greece. A Qualitative Study. *Applied Nursing Research, 53*, 51249. https://doi.org/10.1016/j.apnr.2020.151249
Takechi, H., Sugihara, Y., Matsumoto, H., & Yamada, H. (2018). A dementia café as a bridgehead for community-inclusive care: Qualitative analysis of observations by on-the-job training participants in a dementia cafe. *Dementia and Geriatric Cognitive Disorders, 46*(3–4), 128–139.

Thompson, D. M., Booth, L., Moore, D., & Mathers, J. (2022). Peer support for people with chronic conditions: A systematic review of reviews. *BMC Health Services Research, 22*(1), 427.

Valenzuela-Garcia, H., Molina, J. L., Lubbers, M. J., & Grau, J. (2021). The relational vulnerability of people experiencing multiple exclusion homelessness (MEH) in Spain. *International Journal of Environmental Research and Public Health, 18*, 10275.

VanBronkhorst, S. B., Abraham, E., Dambreville, R., Ramos-Olazagasti, M. A., Wall, M., Saunders, D. C., & Duarte, C. S. (2024). Sociocultural risk and resilience in the context of adverse childhood experiences. *JAMA Psychiatry, 81*(4), 406–413.

Velez, A., & Euronews. (2023). *Tackling social isolation: Northern Europe steps up to the challenge.* Euronews. Retrieved 10 January, 2025 from https://www.euronews.com/my-europe/2023/10/23/tackling-social-isolation-northern-europe-steps-up-to-the-challenge

Victor, C., Scambler, S., & Bond, J. (2008). *EBOOK: The social world of older people: Understanding loneliness and social isolation in later life*. McGraw-Hill Education (UK).

Warren-Jeanpiere, L., Dillaway, H., Hamilton, P., Young, M., & Goparaju, L. (2014). Taking it one day at a time: African American women aging with HIV and co-morbidities. *AIDS Patient Care and STDs, 28*(7), 372–380. https://doi.org/10.1089/apc.2014.0024

Welch, L., Sadler, E., Austin, A., & Rogers, A. (2021). Social network participation towards enactment of self-care in people with chronic obstructive pulmonary disease: A qualitative meta-ethnography. *Health Expectations, 24*(6), 1995–2012. https://doi.org/10.1111/hex.13340

Wellman, B. (2000). Changing connectivity: A future history of Y2.03K. *Sociological Research Online, 4*(4), 171–184.

Weiss, R. S. (1973). *Loneliness: The experience of emotional and social isolation.* The MIT Press.

Willcox, S. (2014). *Chronic diseases in Australia: The case for changing course. Australian Health Policy Collaboration Issues paper No. 2014–02.* Australian Health Policy Collaboration. https://www.vu.edu.au/sites/default/files/chronic-diseases-in-australia-the-case-for-changing-course-mitchell-institute.pdf

Wilson, R., Krueger, K. R., Arnold, S. E., Schneider, J. A., Kelly, J. F., Barnes, L. L., & Bennett, D. A. (2007). Loneliness and Risk of Alzheimer Disease. *Archives of General Psychiatry, 64*(2), 234–240.

Winnicott, D. W. (1958). The capacity to be alone. *The International Journal of Psychoanalysis, 39*, 416–420.
World Health Organisation (WHO). (2025). *WHO Commission on Social Connection.* WHO. Retrieved 10 January, 2025, from https://www.who.int/groups/commission-on-social-connection.
Wright Mills, C. (1959). *The sociological imagination.* Oxford University Press.
Yanguas, J., Pinazo-Henandis, S., & Tarazona-Santabalbina, F. J. (2018). The complexity of loneliness. *Acta Bio Medica: Atenei Parmensis, 89*(2), 302.

2

Insignificant, Irrelevant, and Alienated: Types of Loneliness While Navigating Chronic Illness

Introduction

The onset of a chronic condition requires the individual to reconstruct meaning about their life and their life trajectory. Theorists such as Bury (1982) and Charmaz (1983, 1994, 1995) have described how chronic illness unsettles people's self-identity, body, social roles and the social world through "the disruption of taken-for-granted assumptions and behaviours" (Bury, 1982, p. 169); and that this disruption requires a rethinking of the individual's biography and self-concept (Charmaz, 1983, 1994). In response to disruption, individuals reconstruct and reinterpret the stories of their illness to make sense of their experiences (Frank, 1997). They reconstitute and repair ruptures between body, self and the world, through a process of narrative reconstruction (Williams, 1984). There is also variation in the experience of diagnosis. While for some, the onset of chronic illness is disruptive, for others it is anticipated, expected, minimised, normalised, biographically repaired, and/or affirming (e.g. Sanders et al., 2024).

The narrative meaning-making process in the wake of illness is shaped by both people's social and material embeddedness and culturally available narratives of survivorship, victimhood and suffering (Bigony &

S. Lewis et al., *Unravelling the Layers of Chronic Illness and Loneliness*,
https://doi.org/10.1007/978-981-96-7909-6_2

Keitel, 2020). How people make sense of their experience of illness and the degree to which they experience illness as disruption, is related to their experience of belonging, meaningful social participation, as well as their access to positive representations of living with chronic illness.

How chronic illnesses are socially constructed and interpreted by the self and others are also implicated in the experience of loneliness. Normative understandings of chronic illnesses, which encompass both biomedical classifications and wider social meanings, affect how those with chronic illnesses relate to others and how others respond and relate to them (Sointu, 2016). These understandings are also linked to broader social hierarchies of illness (Album et al., 2017) with some illnesses more widely understood and socially recognised evoking support and sympathy in the public imagination. In contrast, other illnesses, especially many chronic conditions, are less likely to receive empathy or social support. (Stone, 2018). Cultural assumptions and moral judgements about culpability, self-responsibility, obligation and deservedness of care and support comprise societal understanding of chronic illnesses. These understandings can all contribute to the experience of loneliness.

These experiences are particularly evident for people with illnesses that are medically contested (e.g. myalgic encephalomyelitis/chronic fatigue syndrome), evade medical categorisation, lack public or medical recognition, breach social norms and expectations and/or when the person is deemed to have caused their illness through "poor" lifestyle choices (e.g. type 2 diabetes) (Riles et al., 2023). Similarly, where conditions are not visually "readable" (e.g. fibromyalgia, some mental illnesses and autoimmune conditions) (Groenevelt & de Boer, 2023), where symptoms are invisible or not seen as "real", individuals may be denied credibility and may be stereotyped on the basis that they "don't look unwell". As we show in Chapter Four, social bonds can become weakened or tenuous when individuals feel that others misunderstand or invalidate their experience of illness (Lewis et al., 2024a). In these scenarios, people can struggle for legitimacy of their suffering, which in turn can make them feel isolated or marginalised in their experience, as well as socially ostracised by others (Franklin et al., 2019; Lewis et al., 2024b).

As discussed in Chapter One, there are similarities between chronic illness and loneliness in how they are understood and interpreted. Like chronic illness, dominant understandings of loneliness in Western societies such as Australia, locate the causes of loneliness in the individual, for example associating it with a person's lack of social skills or reluctance to participate in social activities. Like chronic illness, loneliness can also be stigmatised (Sagan, 2023). Neves and Petersen (2025) propose that the (largely psychological) literature portrays loneliness as an affliction encountered by "loners" and the "socially inept" (p. 3). In contrast, their sociological study of older Australians suggests that while the stigma of loneliness can lead to personal feelings of shame, pain and guilt, it should be understood as the intersection of personal, social and structural phenomena. They found that the label "lonely" may fuel stereotyping and discrimination in social interactions, and argued that loneliness is often a product of the social system, practices and processes (Neves & Petersen, 2025).

The complexity of the meanings and experiences of loneliness is evident in research showing that loneliness is associated with abandonment and estrangement from meaningful personal relationships and communities, feeling unable to relate to others, feeling trapped or bored, and with limited access to valued activities (Band & Rogers, 2024; Malli et al., 2023). Yet, the meanings and subjective experiences of loneliness for those with chronic illness remain underexplored (see for exception Lewis et al., 2024b; Wotherspoon, 2024). Participants in our research described how they gave meaning to their experience of chronic conditions and loneliness and, importantly, how constructions and experiences of loneliness shape and are shaped by experiences of chronic illness. Their meanings can be categorised into three broad, sometimes overlapping, types of loneliness.

Loneliness as Insignificance: "I'm Too Broken"

Many participants constructed loneliness in terms of their relationship to themselves. Describing loneliness as personal insignificance, they found it difficult to construct positive meaning in their lives. Rather than being primarily attributed to the quality of their relationships with others, this "internal" form of loneliness emerged from participants' self-perceptions as being “different”, “defective” and “faulty”— identities shaped by their experience of physical and/or mental chronic ill-health. Natalia spoke of feeling “broken”, due to a long history of physical and mental health challenges. While she longed to build connections with significant others with whom she could share her life, her fear of being judged or rejected by others was an insurmountable barrier:

> Natalia: I would definitely like to be more connected, but I always hold back. I just find that difficult. I sometimes feel that I don’t know how to connect with people. I’ve just been on my own for so long. And I say to my psychologist quite often, “I’m too broken”. So, letting people in is just something that I find really, really difficult.
>
> Interviewer: When you say “broken”, are you thinking from the past?
>
> Natalia: Just physically and mentally. I feel that I have too many issues and that I would be too challenging for someone and they just wouldn’t stay anyway. It’s a loop that you just end up thinking, “I want somebody, I want to be with someone, I want to share my life with someone,” but doing that and bringing someone into you and your home, the anxiety of that, just I think, “I can’t do that.” (Natalia, 30s, with multiple physical health conditions)

Others similarly described themselves as “unlovable”, “unlikeable” unworthy of affection or felt that they had little to contribute to friendships, groups or society. These beliefs created a negative spiral where loneliness was followed by feelings of self-blame, self-pity and shame, a tendency to become more sensitive to rejection, assumptions that others harboured negative thoughts about them and a lack of trust in the people around them. This spiral in turn worsened feelings of loneliness. Verna, a single woman in her late sixties with multiple sclerosis (MS) articulated this tension well. Verna described a profound sense of aloneness and insignificance that worsened at particular times of year, such as Christmas:

> It’s always sort of lurking. I can even feel tears welling up a bit now. It’s always there, watching television, reading a story. [...] it’s that deep, really

> deep inside. It raises its head, particularly at this time of year. I'm better this year than I have been in previous years. You get really lonely. You think, "I've got no family. I've got no one." And you can go in for a bout of self-pity, which is never really the right track. (Verna, 60s, with MS)

Fear of being shamed or discredited by others meant many participants chose to restrict social activities that they highly valued. Shame and self-rejection also made it difficult to share feelings of loneliness with others and to reach out for support. Michella lived with significant pain due to systemic lupus erythematosus and complications following two hip replacements and a spinal fusion. She described herself as "fiercely independent". She had not disclosed her health condition to friends, family or colleagues, as she feared others would feel responsible or perceive her as a "whiner". Wanting to not be a burden to others, Michella tended to overcompensate by "dragging" herself to work although she was in considerable pain. Even her best friend of 20 years did not know that Michella had systemic lupus erythematosus. Having a chronic condition became, in Michella's words, "a dirty little secret". However, not sharing such a significant part of her life created a disconnect between herself and others. Michella described that, although she might be able to manage the physical pain with the help of pain medication, the emotional pain of loneliness was at times unbearable. In the quote below, Michella discussed how she both felt shame for being lonely and blamed herself for these feelings:

> I always feel that it [loneliness] is sitting in the background. But I'm the one that chooses to have that there. But yeah, it's just that I've done it for so long. And not talking about private life or health issues, like I said, it's all a dirty little secret that you just keep hidden and that just exacerbates everything. It's not wanting people to look at you differently, to discriminate against you or to think, "She's a liability," or to even think, "Well, she might die, so I'm not going to get close to her". […] But again, it's not letting people in and telling them about things. Because you don't want them to think, "Oh god, oh, she's complaining again." You want to try to be a person that people want to be around, but sometimes that's just too damn hard to do. So, it's easier just to sit at home and be in your pain, mentally or physically, rather than invite people in. Because you think

> that once they see the true thing and the true wholeness of it all, that they're not going to want to be involved anyway. So why let somebody in and then be disappointed or heartbroken when they leave? So, it's better just to be alone. (Michella, 50s, with systemic lupus erythematosus)

Despite describing the social and physical conditions that restricted opportunities for their social participation, some participants still perceived loneliness as something within their personal control. Michella captured this idea by attributing loneliness to her decision to not disclose her health issues. She noted that being dependent on others for connection was something to be avoided, a sentiment that many participants shared.

The idea that loneliness was a personal failing or weakness and an issue to be managed by the individual was reinforced in some messages that participants received from their family members or friends. Participants described a fear of being stigmatised by others if they were to disclose that they were lonely. Renee spoke of not wanting to become a burden to her family and thus feeling that she should deal with her loneliness on her own. Seeking connection with others, for her, was a risky endeavour as illustrated here:

> Interviewer: What would happen if you did share those feelings of loneliness?
> Renee: Well, it's really hard because I think they're all so busy, my children. I think they'd probably make a big effort for about a week and then things would get busy again.
> And I don't want them feeling that they've got to hold my hand. It's my life. And, to me, it feels like it's not their responsibility. […] Who can make you happy? You can. I mean, definitely other people can make you happy and your circumstances can. But ultimately, it is you that makes you happy, isn't it? […] You don't want people to think, "Oh god, not her again; "You're going to whinge and moan". (Renee, 70s, with chronic obstructive pulmonary disease (COPD))

Seeing loneliness as an individual concern and responsibility prevented individuals from seeking out support. Some participants avoided disclosing their loneliness to others because they feared it would be trivialised or that its seriousness would be diminished. For example, Adelaide recently moved into a retirement village to be closer to her daughter and grandchildren. Although family members visited Adelaide once a month, the rest of the time she felt lonely and isolated. Adelaide had hoped that by relocating she would become more involved in her daughter's life, imagining that she would be invited for dinners and play an active role in caring for her grandchildren. She was deeply disappointed and hurt that this had not eventuated and felt that most of the responsibility to stay connected with her daughter's family fell on her. Adelaide felt that her daughter would question, trivialise, or minimise her feelings if she was to seek more intimacy from her or disclose that she felt lonely:

> If I didn't do anything, if I said, "No, I'm not going," I don't think anyone would bother. I think I'd be left here. [My family] don't notice. They don't. And if I said anything, they'd say, "What? Go on. Look Mum, you've got this and you've got that and you've got that." You know? They wouldn't believe me. (Adelaide, 80s, with pulmonary fibrosis and osteoporosis)

In seeking to make sense of their experiences, most participants viewed loneliness through a lens of personal failings or intrinsic character flaws. The trivialising, minimising or silencing of their experience of loneliness both in cultural discourses and in conversations with family and friends further reinforced their belief that they should feel ashamed of their loneliness. Consequently, participants constructed loneliness as an experience outside the boundaries of normalcy—and therefore, something to be hidden.

Loneliness as Irrelevance: "Nobody Will Care if I am Here or Not"

A second type of loneliness described by participants occurred in interpersonal encounters and was the absence of recognition or appreciation by others, reinforcing feelings of irrelevance. Participants described loneliness as "not feeling heard or seen", "feeling forgotten" and "not having a connection to somebody who makes you feel like you have inherent value". Being a significant part of someone's life and participating in shared activities was described as important for experiencing a sense of meaning in life. Participants detailed various large and small moments where they had felt important, useful, valued or where they experienced themselves as a part of another person's life or shared a personal moment with them. A recurring feature of participants' stories was that these moments were rare or fleeting occurrences. Thus, for most participants, their loneliness as irrelevance was associated with the longing for more involvement in social life. For example, Nelly yearned for close friends and emotional intimacy and described how her irrelevance was reinforced in a relationship with a "really close" friend:

> I feel lonely, especially if there's something I want to talk to somebody about and you can't talk to them when you want to talk to them about it. I've got a girlfriend who calls in once a week, and we're really close, but for some reason, I go talk to her about something or I want to talk to her about something and she's got to go. And then I don't want to ring her up and bug her on the phone, so I think, "No, look, forget about it." And look, times like that, I feel a little bit lonely. I'd like to talk about something. Yeah, talk to somebody about something. It doesn't matter what it's about. Just, yeah, those times I might feel lonely. (Nelly, 70s, with COPD)

Nelly longed for a connection with others whom she could talk to, confide in, discuss her problems with and ultimately share her world with. Others, who had wider social networks, discussed loneliness as the absence of quality connections. For Betty loneliness arose from the lack of reliable and meaningful friendships and she described her social connections with others as fleeting, superficial or unreliable:

> The word "loneliness", it brings up a very strong feeling inside me, a feeling of sadness, and what that tells me is that there's something there for me about what you're saying. I do feel that lack of connection in my life. So, I think that loneliness is about having that lack of connection, which, for me, I would describe as meaningful and reliable. (Betty, 40s, with chronic pain, musculoskeletal issues and post-traumatic stress disorder (PTSD))

Laura, who lives alone, described her social connections as limited to paid support workers:

> I often feel socially, isolated mentally. I guess physically I'm not, because physically I can find someone probably to have coffee with or, yeah, I can ring a support worker or something. And most days I have a lot of things on. So physically, I'm not isolated as such. Having a mental illness can make you feel very, very lonely because people don't really understand what it's like. So that's how I would describe it, physically not, mentally yes. (Laura, 50s, with arthritis and bipolar disorder)

Similarly, living alone in social housing, with no family support and with neighbours she does not trust, Verna's network was comprised of a team of paid support workers to take her to the park, collect her shopping, and provide her with company and activities around her home. While Verna appreciated the regular social contact, these relationships were organised around her care needs rather than mutual interests or reciprocal connection:

> I have one chap who comes on a Monday and with the help of him and his wife, we've built this really beautiful garden. I have another lady who comes twice a week and we usually go shopping on a Friday or go for a walk... And last year, thanks to my support workers, was the first time I'd been to the beach in 15 years...so I do have a good network. (Verna, 60s, with MS)

For most participants, the onset of a chronic illness or a marked acceleration in physical or mental decline also resulted in a noticeable break from their prior experiences of social connections. Feelings of irrelevance and increased loneliness were evident in participant accounts when they described trying to share their experience with others who could not, or would not, relate to them. Tammy who was diagnosed with MS in her forties, lamented the absence of a shared understanding with friends and her partner:

> This is very egocentric kind of thing, but they can't possibly understand what I'm going through, so what's the point? And that's loneliness. Yeah, because even the closest person to me, he isn't able to get it, because he knows me so well, and better than anyone else, but he will never 100% understand how it feels inside... It feels like there's this unfair level, a very unbalanced level of burden on me to try and have that normal relationship, while I'm dealing with what's going on inside of me, physically and emotionally. [...] So, I think that loneliness is that I can understand how an able-bodied, normal person without MS would feel, because I was that. So, I feel like I have that knowledge. So, look at me, lucky me, I get to know that. And you don't get to know this, so that's mine and mine alone. And rather than feeling special about it, I feel quite isolated by it. I wish I didn't have that. I wish I was just able to just be human like you. (Tammy, 40s, with MS)

Tammy, like many others, described the lingering loneliness following a health crisis, deepened by a heightened awareness of the fragility of connectedness. Having a health crisis, or having one's life completely upturned by an illness, changed participants in ways that were difficult for them to articulate. Although some participants were surrounded by others and continued their customary roles as parents, partners or friends, they described feeling alone in a reality that others did not share—a sense of belonging to a "different world". It was the contrast of the "two worlds", that of illness and that of "normalcy", that exposed the feeling of irrelevance experienced by participants. The severity of disruptions that their condition had brought to their friendships was followed by feelings of loss, grief, pain and frustration.

The absence of similar others who could provide emotional support and validate their identity created what Stein and Solomon (2017) term "loneliness of experiential isolation". This type of loneliness was rooted in the absence of empathic understanding in the face of the magnitude of what they had experienced. Gaining such vital shared understanding, usually through disclosure to others, was described as an antidote to loneliness. However, the act of disclosure was not without risks. Participants relayed encounters with people who judged them or offered advice without understanding the depth of their situation and the profound loneliness this created. Tina discussed such an experience and how it left her feeling misunderstood, shamed and psychologically and emotionally detached. Tina experienced significant mobility issues due to fibromyalgia which meant her abilities, pain level and energy level changed daily:

> I remember reaching out to one of my partner's family members to explain like, "Hey, at that wedding, I know you were very disappointed I couldn't get on the dance floor with you, but I just wasn't feeling well, and it was a real push for me to even come to this wedding. And I feel like I've hidden my pain a lot in your family, so I'm going to explain what my disability is actually like." And I got a whole, long speech back saying that "I was defining myself by my disability, that I'd given up on myself, I was too reliant on others, and I just need to pull myself up by my bootstraps and stop being such a whiner." And I was frightened for five years to talk to her about that, and that's why. So that's why people with disabilities are afraid to actually advocate for themselves because people don't want to hear it. It's an inconvenience to them. (Tina, 30s, with multiple physical and mental chronic conditions)

The sense of invalidation is clear. Tina articulated how the lack of understanding from a family member and the devaluation of her ongoing experience created loneliness. Others discussed similarly isolating occurrences when people, instead of seeking to understand, offered advice about how to individually fix feelings of loneliness through doing particular activities or adjusting their mindset. This also related to health advice, as Nicola recounted:

> I remember getting a text message from someone. [...] And their advice was, and I really hope at some point I will forget this, but their advice was to become very vegan and to practise the act of gratitude to every single person. And they knew that that worked for MS because they saw it on a YouTube video. And they sent me this video, and I just haven't been able to reply to that. That was a year ago. Because all I wanted to say was really bad words. I just thought, "How can you think that that's a reasonable thing to say to someone on any day of the week anyway." But just, no. Drinking bicarb water, is not going to flush out—You can't piss out MS. I mean, I'm not a urologist, but I'm pretty sure that that's not how it works. So it's just people who just are severely uneducated, but they think they're right. But that, to me, the bit that's challenging is that you can't reason with some of these people and the way that they communicate. So it's like, "You know what? Yep, I'll take isolation. That's okay." (Nicola, 30s, with MS)

Experiences of not feeling listened to and understood also happened in encounters with health staff. These encounters involved not being acknowledged beyond one's health or mental health issues. In instances when healthcare professionals did not have time to engage in meaningful dialogue, some participants recounted feeling treated as objects (Karhe & Kaunonen, 2015). Nicola discussed how her experiences of loneliness were exacerbated when she felt that healthcare providers neither understood nor sought to understand the unique meaning of her experience. Her quote below illustrates the process of disconnectedness that can occur in the absence of genuine connection in encounters between patients and healthcare staff:

> It's very hard to get a genuine connection with people who do not have the slightest idea what the condition is. [...] So, even neurologists, medical specialists, sometimes I just look at them and I think, "Fuck me, you just don't get the whole picture." Sometimes it's like, even with profoundly intelligent or smart people, that can actually be quite lonely as well because everything is based on some sort of agenda. It's not a real human connection. [...] It's a gamble, I think, when you try and connect with people. It's like, "Do I waste my time speaking in a language that just isn't going to be understood?" So, it's a little bit like, "Do I even bother?" (Nicola, 30s, with MS)

Loneliness as Alienation: "The Circle of my Life Has Gotten Smaller and Smaller"

Participants described a third type of loneliness closely related to the experience of chronic illness: alienation from society. This form of loneliness involved a feeling of fundamental separateness from others and the wider world. Participants described a sense of thwarted belongingness, a being "on the sidelines", and being unable to "find a slot to fit into" (see also Lewis et al., 2024b). Being without others and their fellowship was characterised by Laura as observing rather than actively participating in her life:

> I could technically get through a whole week of my life never talking to anyone... I wouldn't have to go anywhere or do anything at all and no one would notice at all. I could probably do that for a month or two. That's not a good thing. That's not right. That's me not being part of the world I'm living in. (Laura, 50s, with arthritis and bipolar disorder)

Laura's excerpt reveals a struggle to find her "fit" within the community, and the vulnerability and shame of her outsider position. Bianca's account similarly illustrates loneliness as alienation. Bianca lives with chronic pain and chronic fatigue caused by fibromyalgia as well as significant autoimmune issues associated with chemical and food intolerances. Her condition requires her to be vigilant when going out as chemicals added to everyday products such as perfume, cleaning products, or air fresheners can make her very ill. She described how the need for vigilance around such exposures had gradually isolated her and made it increasingly difficult for her to undertake activities such as going to the office, to the movies or out for dinner. This sense of loneliness was derived from her inability to participate in society in a meaningful way:

> The last few years have disconnected me from joining in. I'm on the outer. Kind of on the outer. I can't seem to get in the group settings like I used to be. (Bianca, 60s, with fibromyalgia and severe food and chemical sensitivities)

Bianca went on to talk about trying to "rebuild my character to be able to be like I used to be, more social". However, her attempts to find a new way to meaningfully participate in society, added to the intensive and invisible labour that Bianca needed to do in managing her illness. This highlights the limits of overly simplistic "reach out" messaging that encourages lonely individuals to be more engaged in social activities as a remedy to their loneliness. Bianca articulated how the social embeddedness of loneliness manifested through feeling peripheral and unimportant to her social group, and by extension, to greater society. Life seemed meaningless when participants felt that they were unable to contribute or feel important to others, and by extension felt that they did not have a valued social role or identity. Loneliness as social alienation was associated with limited social integration, inability to participate in the labour market and having a disabled body. Not being able to pursue one's vocation or participate in a book club or sporting activities left participants with a reduced feeling of relevance (described above) and belonging. Adelaide discussed how loneliness slowly seeped into her life in step with her dwindling opportunities for participation. She described her previous working life when she felt intrinsically part of communities around work and her interests and contrasted this with the need to actively pursue communities to counter her sense of isolation:

> Because working was like a social network with me, and so I didn't need so much in the social outside because I'd go to work every day and say hello to people and have a chat and go to the Christmas parties or whatever. And so, that's also something you just come to terms with. For some people, like what was happening with me, because I recognised, was that I was becoming reclusive. It wasn't an overnight thing, and even though I've got some people that I can contact, but it's not a weekly or a monthly thing. It was becoming a six-monthly thing. Because it seemed that my world was shrinking so much that I wasn't making those connections. (Adelaide, 80s, with pulmonary fibrosis and osteoporosis)

For many, having a body with reduced capabilities meant they had diminished accessibility to shops or locations that had previously been important and familiar. Ida, retired and in her sixties, related that since her children had moved away, the incidental social connections that she made throughout the day with people in her local community had been a much-valued source of social connection. However, losing her mobility due to MS cut her off from these casual acquaintances as she could no longer visit shops or cafes on her own, intensifying her sense of community exclusion:

> I can't go into the shops down here because I can't get into them. I go in with my sister and she helps me. But I used to know people in the town when Luna, my daughter's grown up now, when she was at school, but you lose contact with them because your kids have grown up and moved away. (Ida, 60s, with MS)

Ida's account illustrates the connection between loneliness and social exclusion. For Ida, connection and belongingness were associated with places in her town that facilitated social encounters and group membership. It also illustrates the importance of incidental or casual acquaintances (e.g. shop keepers, neighbours) as valuable sources of social support for those with illness (Moreton et al., 2023). At the time of the interviews, Ida was largely homebound. Losing her independence and ability to choose how she spent her days meant both a loss of choice and agency but also limited opportunities to pursue spaces of belonging and connection as she could before. Instead, Ida now watched life continue outside her window without feeling able to participate:

> I used to love to go for a walk. I used to walk every day. And I had a gym membership. I used to like to go to the gym. Now I've got a walker at the back door. I'm flat out to get the paper in the morning. And everybody walks past my house, walking their dog and jogging. You think, "You're so lucky." Yeah, they're so lucky. [Before] I was totally independent, my own person. I did what I wanted. If I wanted to nick here or nick there, you'd go there. You could just do whatever you wanted to do, whatever you felt like doing. Yeah, you just can't go anywhere. The circle of my life has got smaller and smaller. I used to have a big wide circle, went to work and went places and everything. Now my circle's just getting smaller and smaller. (Ida, 60s, with MS)

A shrinking life and shrinking social circle due to chronic illness were described in many interviews. Participants relayed how the dwindling of their life was both an external and an internal process, a reaction to changing life situations, to losing previous abilities and independence, but also an emotional experience of increasing vulnerability, unsafety, hopelessness and not wanting to be confronted with physical losses. Michael, semi-retired and in his eighties, previously had a double lung transplant, but had since developed chronic bronchitis, and often needed to use an oxygen tank due to reduced lung capacity. Michael also experienced difficulty walking and fear of falling. Michael described how the vulnerability brought on by his mobility issues, combined with episodes of incontinence, made leaving familiar places both demanding and nerve-wracking. Where previously Michael and his wife enjoyed going out to dinner, cinema or a show, these types of outings became more and more difficult. Often Michael preferred to stay home:

> My wife loves live theatre. There's a show just come to town and she wanted to go, but I said, "I'm just not up to it." So she's going with one of her girlfriends, and I'm happy with that. To save all the hassles, I'll drive the two girls there and pick them up later, but I won't go to the show. I'd love to see it, but I just couldn't handle the steps and the crowds. It's my life with my breathing problems. I'm on diuretics, right, and at the moment I'm taking pretty heavy, severe, large doses of diuretics, which means I'm running to the toilet to wee just about all the time. And I'm just thinking to myself, "Oh, if I go to the cinema or go to the theatre, in the middle of the show I've got to get up." I thought, "Oh, it's just not worth the effort." Also, going to the cinema or a theatre with a walker or a crutch and going upstairs and then in the middle of the show and I just—Maybe I'm being a bit of a coward, I don't know, but I just don't fancy the idea of having to be confronted with that situation… My world has shrunk in the last few months by virtue of the fact that I'm limited with my activities. (Michael, 80s, with complications from a double lung transplant)

For Michael, alienation was not associated with particular places themselves, but with his diminished ability to master and navigate such places. Other participants discussed how their loneliness was exacerbated when they were confronted by mainstream societies' lack of accommodation for people with different abilities. They described their efforts to "fit in" to a world that was not built for them. Struggling with opening doors, entering buildings or accessing items in the supermarket brought to the forefront a sense of exclusion from the mainstream. This sense of loneliness brought on by feeling disabled was exacerbated by the actions of others. Nicola discussed her observations of the widespread lack of consideration from others in the community towards people living with illness. Seeing the lack of accommodation afforded to others with special needs confronted Nicola with her own sense of difference and brought on a sense of loneliness. This loneliness can be said to be associated with feeling excluded from communal spaces:

> There's like this little reminder that you don't fit in. And that, I think, is the real loneliness aspect. I was going to say I don't really care about fitting in, but I think it's more like just not being ostracised. I am an introvert. In a group setting, I'd be finding a way to leave. But sometimes it just feels like there's something printed on my forehead that's like, "Hello, I'm different." So, it's a little bit shit. And then even seeing things, like on public transport, when people are sitting in disabled seats. The other day, I saw a man, an elderly man who was blind, he had a stick and I'm like, "Why the fuck don't people get up?" And so then I'm trying to help him. It was just like, things like that. And even where things are positioned, it's only positioned for mainstream society. (Nicola, 30s, with MS)

Loneliness as alienation was experienced as being untethered from everyone and everything, being abandoned and neglected by mainstream society. Many described such underlying feelings of alienation brought on by living in a physical world mainly catering to the able-bodied community. Participants like Michael, Nicola and Ida highlighted how heightened vulnerability and extended periods of being homebound dovetailed to exacerbate loneliness and social isolation. Feelings of loneliness, inclusion, or exclusion were associated both with the accessibility of the external local environment but also with the extent to which they felt able to meaningfully participate in the world they lived in.

Conclusion

In this chapter, we have illustrated the complexities of loneliness as it is understood and experienced in the everyday lives of those with chronic illness. The types of loneliness experienced by participants with chronic illness occurred at three different relational levels. First, relationship to self, loneliness was perceived as insignificance and a private failing for which personal responsibility is required. Second, in relation to others, loneliness was perceived as irrelevant, arising from feeling unheard, unsupported and invalidated, reinforced when attempts to reach out to others were unsuccessful. Finally, at the societal level, loneliness was perceived as alienation from society and evident in a shrinking social presence and social exclusion (see also Lewis et al., 2024b). Identifying the different types of loneliness and how they are experienced in relation to chronic illness helps us understand diverse social, psychological and contextual issues that are linked to loneliness in people's lives. These types of loneliness are nested within each other, compounding, interacting and overlapping. The feeling of not being understood or seen, coupled with a sense that their illness and loneliness were often not treated with empathy, left participants feeling untethered from the collective.

That loneliness was closely tied with feeling overlooked, diminished, invalidated, misread or misunderstood, demonstrates how cultural mis/understandings or social stigmatisation of different chronic illnesses (especially rare, contested, invisible or multiple chronic conditions) are implicated in loneliness (Groenevelt & de Boer, 2023; Wotherspoon, 2024). These notions extend social science scholarship on how struggles for recognition and legitimisation of the chronic illness create loneliness and other forms of social suffering, such as entrapment, social withdrawal and the severing of social bonds (Broom et al., 2015; Lewis et al., 2024a). Recognition not only related to feeling acknowledged, understood and validated by others, but also to the sense that one both has value and is valued and respected by others. The uncertainty and enduring nature of the conditions affecting participants—their messiness and unpredictability—along with the multiple chronic conditions that many participants described worked against connectedness.

Participant stories of feeling misread, forgotten, and feeling that the world is not made for them, highlight the fallacy of characterisations of loneliness as an individual failing or as social deficiency (discussed in Chapter One). Moreover, these stories reveal how the dominant rhetoric of loneliness as a "problem" of the individual's creation (and remediation) can oversimplify a complex social experience (Sagan, 2023). The shame and stigma of being lonely is amplified while the experience of being lonely (and the work involved in managing both chronic illness and loneliness) is rendered invisible, thus serving to prevent those who experience loneliness from seeking social support. In trying to remedy loneliness in the context of chronic illness, it is important to challenge stigmatising discourse and harmful assumptions ascribed to chronic illness that fuel loneliness. This requires ensuring that public understandings are informed by lived experience. It is also important to understand how ableism limits opportunities for social valuing and inclusion, fuelling the downward spiral of snowballing loneliness and isolation (Malli et al., 2023) as individuals become further separated from community.

References

Album, D., Johannessen, L. E., & Rasmussen, E. B. (2017). Stability and change in disease prestige: A comparative analysis of three surveys spanning a quarter of a century. *Social Science & Medicine, 180*, 45–51.

Band, R., & Rogers, A. (2024). Understanding the meaning of loneliness and social engagement for the workings of a social network intervention connecting people to resources and valued activities. *Health Expectations, 27*(6), Article e70111.

Bigony, C. E., & Keitel, M. A. (2020). Chapter 7—Meaning-making and chronic illness: Understanding through narratives. In E. M. Altmaier (Ed.), *Navigating life transitions for meaning* (pp. 107–127). Academic Press.

Broom, A. F., Kirby, E. R., Adams, J., & Refshauge, K. M. (2015). On illegitimacy, suffering and recognition: A diary study of women living with chronic pain. *Sociology, 49*(4), 712–731.

Bury, M. R. (1982). Chronic illness as biographical disruption. *Sociology of Health and Illness, 18*, 220–240.

Charmaz, K. (1983). Loss of self: A fundamental form of suffering in the chronically ill. *Sociology of Health and Illness, 5*(2), 168–195.

Charmaz, K. (1994). Identity dilemmas of chronically ill men. *The Sociological Quarterly, 35*(2), 69–288. https://doi.org/10.4135/9781452243757.n13

Charmaz, K. (1995). The body, identity, and self: Adapting to impairment. *The Sociological Quarterly, 36*(4), 657–680. https://doi.org/10.1111/j.1533-8525.1995.tb00459.x

Frank, A. W. (1997). *The wounded storyteller—Body, illness, and ethics* (2nd ed.). The University of Chicago Press.

Franklin, M., Lewis, S., Willis, K., Rogers, A., Venville, A., & Smith, L. (2019). Goals for living with a chronic condition: The relevance of temporalities, dispositions, and resources. *Social Science & Medicine, 233*, 13–20.

Groenevelt, I. I., & de Boer, M. M. (2023). Contesting misrecognition online: Experiences of epistemic in/justice by vloggers with contested illnesses. *Social Science & Medicine, 327*, Article 115951.

Karhe, L., & Kaunonen, M. (2015). Patient experiences of loneliness: An evolutionary concept analysis. *Advances in Nursing Science, 38*(4), E21–E34. https://doi.org/10.1097/ANS.0000000000000096

Lewis, S., Newton, G., Kenny, K., & Boyle, F. (2024a). The incurable self: Negotiating social bonds and dis/connection with metastatic breast cancer. *Sociology of Health & Illness, 46*(2), 295–314.

Lewis, S., Willis, K., Smith, L., Dubbin, L., Rogers, A., Lindegaard Moensted, M., & Smallwood, N. (2024b). There but not really involved: The meanings of loneliness for people with chronic illness. *Social Science & Medicine, 343*, Article 116596. https://doi.org/10.1016/j.socscimed.2024.116596

Malli, M. A., Ryan, S., Maddison, J., & Kharicha, K. (2023). Experiences and meaning of loneliness beyond age and group identity. *Sociology of Health & Illness, 45*(1), 70–89.

Mellor, D., Stokes, M., Firth, L., Hayashi, Y., & Cummins, R. (2008). Need for belonging, relationship satisfaction, loneliness, and life satisfaction. *Personality and Individual Differences, 45*, 213–218. https://doi.org/10.1016/j.paid.2008.03.020

Moreton, J., Kelly, C. S., & Sandstrom, G. M. (2023). Social support from weak ties: Insight from the literature on minimal social interactions. *Social and Personality Psychology Compass, 17*(3), Article e12729. https://doi.org/10.1111/spc3.12729

Neves, B., & Petersen, A. (2025). The social stigma of loneliness: A sociological approach to understanding the experiences of older people. *The Sociological Review, 73*(2), 362–383. https://doi.org/10.1177/00380261231212

Riles, J. M., Adams, K., & Davis, W. M. (2023). Culpability framing influences on community support for those managing illness: A multi-malady comparison of mediated health stigma. *Health Communication, 39*(3), 439–450. https://doi.org/10.1080/10410236.2023.2168351

Sagan, O. (2023). Organised loneliness and its discontents. *Diversity & Inclusion Research, 1*(1), Article e12008. https://doi.org/10.1002/dvr2.12008

Sanders, T., Fryer, K., Greco, M., Mooney, C., Deary, V., & Burton, C. (2024). Explanation for symptoms and biographical repair in a clinic for persistent physical symptoms. *SSM Qual Res Health, 5*, Article 100438. https://doi.org/10.1016/j.ssmqr.2024.100438

Sointu, E. (2016). Discourse, affect and affliction. *Sociological Review, 64*(2), 312–328.

Stein, J. Y., & Solomon, Z. (2017). The lonely side of war's aftermath: Traumatization and isolation among veterans. In O. Sagan & E. Miller (Eds.), *Narratives of loneliness: Multidisciplinary perspectives from the 21st century* (pp. 35–47). Routledge.

Stone, L. (2018). Disease prestige and the hierarchy of suffering. *Medical Journal of Australia, 208*(2), 60–62.

Williams, G. (1984). The genesis of chronic illness: Narrative re-construction. *Sociology of Health & Illness, 6*(2), 175–200.

Wotherspoon, N. (2024). Compelled loneliness and necessitated social isolation: "It's like being on the other side of a mirror, just looking in." *Sociology of Health & Illness, 46*(4), 744–761.

3

"The Life I Should Have Lived": The Significance of Time in Experiencing Chronic Illness and Loneliness

Introduction

Chronic illness directly challenges, for most, normative approaches to understanding linear life course expectations which prescribe how "one should transition from child to adult, find a partner, get married, reproduce, work, eventually transition from adulthood to old age, retire and die" (Ljuslinder et al., 2020, p. 37). The onset of a chronic illness can profoundly shift how time is experienced, understood and spent. The unpredictability of chronic illness disturbs life rhythms and thus, how the past, present and future are constructed and experienced (Harrison et al., 2024). This creates a disjuncture between past/healthy and present/ill selves (Bury, 1982) and, as shown in Chapter Two, alienation from society. Having shared routines, achieving milestones, and participating in significant life events are important (yet often imperceptible) sources of belonging for people, providing vital temporal markers that tether them to their communities. This belonging is often taken for granted and does not become noticeable until it is disrupted. It is not until a person finds themselves "off time": that is, out of step with their peers or significant others, or when they are not progressing through their life in

S. Lewis et al., *Unravelling the Layers of Chronic Illness and Loneliness*, https://doi.org/10.1007/978-981-96-7909-6_3

a linear, forward-moving way, that they feel marginalised from the "social clock" (May, 2008).

Chronic illness involves negotiating an ever-changing temporality in relation to clock and lived time; rather than predictable and linear, time becomes "broken" and unpredictable (Cluley et al., 2024). Managing a chronic illness often means living with oscillating energy levels, pain and fatigue. When individuals' capacities slow down or are reduced due to illness, there may be a need for the slowing down of time to enable opportunities for care and rest. Everyday activities may take longer than usual or require more rest breaks, challenging normative societal expectations about being productive. Social expectations to be spontaneous can also be impacted by the demands and unpredictability of chronic illness as flexibility and freedom associated with being healthy are reduced. Additionally, managing illness is time-consuming, reshaping lives and, in some cases, the lives of carers through the structuring of health-related activities. The need to adhere to medication and dietary regimens, attend regular doctors' appointments and maintain other self-care routines can restrict the person's capacity for improvisation and spontaneity; their life must orientate around a new illness-focused time-schedule (Morris, 2008; see also Cluley et al., 2024). These time-consuming health-related activities can, in turn, hold the person hostage to time-sensitive illness management or what Morris (2008) refers to as "chronic time". The more time that is spent attending to illness-related activities, the less time available to participate in social events and activities. Thus, time can be simultaneously experienced as dragging, speeding up and being taken away. Cluley et al. (2024) argue, with regard to patients receiving dialysis, the lengthening of time and simultaneous reduced capacity for everyday activities "conflicts with the normative expectations embedded within clock time and life-course perspectives" (p. 24).

The interplay of past, present and future time is also pertinent to understanding experiences of loneliness and belonging. May (2017), in her research with older people, found that loneliness in later life can be ameliorated through contemplating a past time when the person felt more socially connected (see also May & Muir, 2015; Routledge et al., 2012). Conversely, past experiences of loneliness can accompany the person into their present lives and can be projected outwards into the future, as we illuminate below. Individuals with chronic illness, especially those who also experience social disadvantage or marginalisation, can experience a loss of a sense of the future and their place within it. Feelings of hope and optimism for the future are important in promoting agency and, in turn, can act as a powerful antidote to loneliness in the present. However, chronic illness can heighten one's awareness of their own bodily restrictions and mortality, and potentially curtail their hopes and aspirations (Alacovska, 2018). Insights from participants in our research show how time is implicated in their experiences of loneliness (see also Cheung et al., 2025). Below, we show how time, chronic illness and experiences of loneliness intersect as participants describe feeling left behind by their peers, the disruption of anticipated life events, and how past experiences of loneliness and loss intrude in the present, contributing to uncertainty about the future.

Left Behind and Losing Life's Map

Participants described how chronic illnesses necessitated a slowing down of the pace and regularity of social activities, particularly when compared with their life before diagnosis. Adapting to the ever-changing demands of the body involved living out of step and out of time with the world of others. Time became constricted as fatigue and pain required participants to ration their energy, limiting what could be done in a day, while mental strain affected their ability to follow conversations and participate in groups. The volatility and fluctuation associated with many chronic illnesses unsettled important dimensions of time, such as the predictability, rhythms and linearity of life. Nicola, recently diagnosed with multiple sclerosis (MS) described, across her three interviews, that loneliness was tied to feeling unable to keep up with societal expectations about pace of life, productivity and how much one could (or should) do each day. Her illness had enforced a change of job—from a fast-paced, high-pressure corporate position—to a part-time book-keeping role. Her quote below illustrates how illness amplified an incongruence between clock time and lived time, as well as the struggles of prioritising and legitimising time for rest and self-care:

> That's kind of where I blame myself a bit, because in no way had I even remotely factored in this [being diagnosed with MS] possibly happening…I didn't have the strategies to deal with anything like this in the first place. I didn't have the work life balance, I didn't have a, I don't know, real ability to do not much during a day. I always had to be doing something, to be achieving something. And I still, even every day, I kind of think, "I wonder what I can get away with today?" Like I'm some horrible real estate agent to myself where I'm like, "How can I sell this?" as if that could convince my central nervous system to be different. (Nicola, 30s, with MS)

For Nicola and many other participants, work had been vital to social cohesion and self- and social worth; it was where participants forged friendships, found purpose and meaningful contribution (Henning, 2017). In a society that privileges productivity and financial and other work-related forms of citizenship, the loss of the ability to work, and in some cases, the need to be on government benefits (e.g. disability support pensions or unemployment benefits), left many participants feeling valueless. As shown in Chapter Two, these changes in how participants felt about self (their worth and their abilities) was central to their experiences of loneliness. Few participants were able to work full-time. Not being able to participate in employment created a sense of being disconnected from a valued aspect of life, leaving some participants more isolated and confined to the home. Participants also described how illness had impacted their ability to fully engage in valued social activities such as physical activity, work performance, being a good friend or being a valuable member of the community:

> I used to walk a lot. I was not a sporting person or anything like that, but I used to do a lot of things. I studied full-time and worked part-time and I was the kind of person that would park in the far away parking space and walk… And now it's like I can't do those kinds of things anymore. (Natalia, 30s, with multiple physical health conditions)

> I feel people look down on [me] which I've never felt before, especially as a professional. I always felt respected in my workplace, a team player in my workplace, and a leader in my workplace. I don't feel that actually,

> when you live with chronic pain. Because you can't participate, you're not productive. Yeah, what can you give back to the community? (Eloise, 60s, with rare neurological autoimmune condition and other chronic conditions)

Participants also shared that loneliness was associated with feeling forgotten or left behind, resulting in a sense of being stranded or stuck in time while they watched their peers move forward on a conventional (linear) life course. They witnessed peers accomplish significant milestones like finding a partner, progressing their career, or becoming a parent, often seemingly with ease. Seeing others accomplish these milestones could generate unwanted feelings of resentment or jealousy of others' lives. Participants described how they increasingly found it difficult to sympathise with the "mundane" issues of their friends, while their own lives had become epitomised by struggle that was difficult for them to share. The inability to keep up with peers and achieve what they wanted for their lives is illustrated by Natalia and Rosemary:

> I'm in a position in my life where I should be able to do stuff and enjoy myself, but because of my condition, I can't. (Natalia, 30s, with multiple physical health conditions)

> I was working, I was the bread winner, and I loved my job. I was a youth worker and I intended to do some more study and do some more professional development and enhance that role. And I had my network of work friends, and then all of a sudden that just changed and I was back home, not driving. And that's been a real journey and a battle. Just readapting to life as it is now. It's been up and down and had different aspects to it. And I've still made new friends and done things, but just not doing the things that I wanted to do at this age. I'd have been retired now and doing things that retired people do, but I'm not. (Rosemary, 60s, with a tick-borne disease and progressive gait disorder)

Being unable to achieve valued cultural milestones or rites of passage that anchored people in time, as Rosemary describes above, created a sense of being untethered or cut adrift not only from peers, but also from pre-illness life and imagined futures.

The experience of temporal derailment from all dimensions of "normal" (pre-illness) life is articulated by Tammy. Before becoming ill, Tammy could not recall feeling lonely or disconnected, having always had good friends and a close relationship with her two sisters. She reflected that in the past, she had only experienced loneliness fleetingly, at moments "where I didn't have plans for the weekend". She commented: "I never really felt lonely outside of that" and "I've never really felt out of place or out of touch prior to this". For Tammy, loneliness was associated with lost relatability with her peers and having life and life plans derailed by illness. Her experience highlights how the collective rhythms of others based around traditional notions of time, including the weekend as leisure time, can pervade the experiences of people with chronic illness. Disentangling oneself from others' temporalities, such as shared expectations of life progression held within one's closest social circle, became a painful point of comparison about what had been lost:

> They're the closest comparison I have to what my life was or what it could be. …Their reality is what mine would have been. So that's quite hard. (Tammy, 40s, with MS)

Tammy described the impact of MS as marked and sudden, affecting her ability to perform her work duties, and ultimately forcing her to change jobs: "I couldn't do that job and it was clear. I was making quite a lot of mistakes". Tammy also described no longer being able to participate in the leisure activities she previously enjoyed, such as bushwalking, mountain biking, and her book club. Like meaningful work, these valued leisure pursuits had been important in anchoring her in time and space, providing a sense of comfort and secure identity. She described the impact of failing mobility and energy levels on physical and other social activities:

> It did really change my ability to socialise. I was in book groups, and I just don't have it in me to go and sit and discuss books late at night now. It's very much impacted my, it's changed how I live my social life, for sure. … I don't have the energy, after using my mind all day, to then go and actually try and exercise later in the evenings. And definitely, if I

> tried to exercise in the morning, I wouldn't be able to get myself to work. It's a strange thing, because the more I use my mind, the weaker my body is, and if I use my body too much, my mind is a bit foggy. (Tammy, 40s, with MS)

The temporal dimension of loneliness is demonstrated in Tammy's description of being left behind by friends due to her limited capacity to participate in social events. Tammy described how the sense of lost relatability left her feeling lonely, as she was now mainly limited to socialise with people who were at different points in their lives (older people or young mothers); and this increased the imperative for her to remain in the paid workforce, even at a reduced capacity:

> I had certain groups of friends that kind of dropped away after I was diagnosed. People didn't understand it or found it too close to home because they were my contemporaries. And then I was home, and it's not healthy to be alone like that. And I was surrounded by either the aged, who were the only other people around, or the non-working mums that I didn't really relate to that well anyway. So, it was important for me to get back to work to socialise, but also to feel like I'm contributing. Actually, a lot of self-worth is wrapped up in my career. (Tammy, 40s, with MS)

Regardless of the efforts or affordances made by others, socialising served as a constant reminder of what Tammy could no longer do. These social comparisons constrained her ability to connect with friends and created a deep sense of shame and fear of others' judgement. Her chronic illness introduced embodied constraints as well as a temporal loneliness into her life, curtailing her life trajectory. This feeling of temporal unbelonging was especially heightened in her relationships with her sisters. It was the lost relatability and shared life path with them, she lamented most:

> There's been lots of things in our lives that are unique, but we all got married and we all had children and we all kind of reached those life milestones, at different points, but we all got there. So, they're all things we can relate to each other. We all had the same parents that split and supported each other through that. And we've all had different illnesses and things have come and gone that way. But they haven't had this, and

> this isn't one of those things that you just have and you work through it and it goes away. This is something that stays there and bounces up and down all the time and throws up stuff and throws curve balls. And that's something they can't get, they can't relate to. (Tammy, 40s, with MS)

Intrusive Pasts

The past was an intrusive presence featuring in many participants' experiences of loneliness and was experienced as grief and longing for what had been lost. Participants discussed longing for their previous life when they could spontaneously meet up with friends and evocatively described a previous ease of enjoyment of life's activities, the outdoors or their social network. Longing for what had been lost included previous identities (e.g. "I was a party girl', "I was a musician"); lost capabilities ("I can't go out alone", "I can't travel', "I cannot work"); and lost opportunities for meaningful social participation ("I used to play bridge", "I was part of a book club", "I was part of a swimming team"). Participants associated the past with nostalgia and reminiscence about a time filled with more connections, avenues of belonging and the capacity to participate in life. At the same time, for some, thoughts of the past were bitter-sweet, filled with reminders of people and places long lost, an arena filled with regrets and missed opportunities, as well as a source of warm memories. Luke, in his late sixties and living with visual impairment, multiple health issues and severe chronic pain, described loneliness as most acute when he thought about his estrangement from his brother and sister. Luke returned again and again during the interviews to the lost closeness and love he had experienced as a child when he was still in contact with his siblings. As he described:

> My sister, when I was a child, she's four years older than me, going to school I remember her holding my hand so I could cross streets. She'd have my school bag. And my brother, he did things. I miss all that. I do. … it would be lovely to have my sister or my brother or both of them. […] Yeah. And I miss them. I miss them. I miss them terribly. And not just them. I miss my nephews… It's a different loneliness. See, if I don't

> speak to my friends about my health, et cetera, that's fine. But I used to confide in my siblings, and I can't anymore. And maybe, I don't know, maybe I've confided in them too much that they couldn't cope with all my health problems. (Luke, 60s, with visual impairment, chronic pain and other chronic conditions)

For participants like Luke, reminiscing still held meaning but was also a reminder of lost connections. This was especially the case for people who were older or who were diagnosed with a chronic illness later in life. Some participants were able to look back at a life well-lived, the past experienced as a source of belonging and a remedy to current loneliness. For others the past, rather than being a source of comfort, was described as a lonely place. Participants with histories of trauma and loneliness had in many cases come to rely on themselves and developed coping mechanisms such as seeking solitude and connections with non-human sources of connection, like nature and other animals (as we discuss in more detail in Chapters Four and Five). Betty, whose experiences of loneliness were associated with trauma and being unsafe, described seeking solitude as a means of protecting herself from further relational danger. As Betty's quote illustrates, trauma and loneliness were braided together in the past and persisted in the present:

> I don't feel like I received physical and verbal affection. I know I was lonely and angry. I journaled. Sometimes I would sit in the library at lunchtime by myself and read. I read a lot. I loved fantasy. It was an escape for me. (Betty, 40s, with chronic pain, musculoskeletal issues and post-traumatic stress disorder (PTSD))

Childhood trauma was discussed by some participants as a way the past continued to instil a sense of loneliness into the present. Similar to Betty, Ross also highlighted how a lifetime of loneliness casts long shadows. Ross described how childhood trauma created enduring loneliness. Seeking to flee this feeling, he adopted a gregarious persona, going to the pub every night and keeping constantly busy. Although his loneliness remained largely hidden from his friends, Ross described an underlying vulnerability, that would show itself when challenges arose:

> I mean, most of my life I used to feel so freaking lonely, it was terrible. That's how I felt. I couldn't stay home alone. Look, when I lived on my own, I used to go up to the club every night. And because I've got that circle of friends, and I can have a fun time with people, people probably wouldn't realise the real me. So I'm fun and I'm having friends and all that and I go home and then I would stay busy working, painting houses all day. And then, if I came to that point, where I didn't have a partner or I didn't have anyone, I would be super, super unbearably lonely. If something went wrong in my life, like if a relationship broke down, it'd impact me way too much. I'd be mortified. I'd be crying. (Ross, 60s, with arthritis and chronic back pain)

The past held no refuge for people with traumatic experiences in childhood or a lifetime of hardship and disadvantage. The association between childhood trauma and adult loneliness is well-established (Hyland et al., 2019). Childhood trauma is associated with depression and anxiety in adulthood, which can affect individuals' ability to socialise and form meaningful relationships in adulthood. The extracts above highlight the difficulties people with trauma experienced forming meaningful relationships across the life course. These difficulties were compounded by chronic illness.

Yet it was not just the past that impacted on how loneliness was experienced in the present. While participants described how their past experiences of not belonging or disconnection played out in the present, these histories also shaped expectations for future social connectivity, creating a sense of pessimism or trepidation about what the future might hold, as we detail in the next section.

Stolen Futures

Past and present experiences of illness, loneliness, and loss, in turn affected how participants viewed and planned for their future. Participants reported fearing for the future because of their worries about managing symptoms and pain, and what that would mean for their social support and social connectedness. We return to the experience of Tammy to exemplify the notion of "stolen futures". Tammy, like many other participants, perceives her past and present through a future she is denied, describing a longing for the "life I should have lived". Her loneliness was associated with feeling robbed of the life she had envisioned for herself. Although the physicality of life had changed for Tammy since illness, her values and understanding of a good life, and how to achieve this, had not. Her visions for the future were, however, largely unattainable now.

Having life insurance and owning their house, Tammy and her husband were able to "future-proof the house" by making it disability and wheelchair friendly. This allowed Tammy a temporary sense of agency and control in feeling prepared for the future. However, at the time of the second interview, Tammy had experienced an exacerbation of her symptoms and was struggling to come to terms with her new circumstances. Tammy had lost considerable mobility and now relied on walking aids and the assistance of a carer to leave the house. Tammy described feeling cut off from the life she had imagined for herself and the future she had looked forward to:

> When I was diagnosed initially, it's a great reprioritising, you shift everything that you felt was important and that perspective completely, irrevocably changed. So, now it's kind of throwing that back at me again. Because I had really felt a false sense of security in where I was going with my condition, thinking, "This is great. The kids are older, I can get back to what I love doing more of." But that's not so much the case… I actually really saw it in my life plan that, as my kids got to this age, one at school and the other one nearly finishing school soon, well a year and a bit, that I would be able to work full-time and really get back into a career. So, I was pretty angry about what that meant to me. (Tammy, 40s, with MS)

While Tammy had the material resources available to try and prepare for the future, for other participants, future planning had lost its meaning due to a sense of overwhelming uncertainty and as a reaction to the limited choices available. These participants disregarded or feared the future because they lacked hope for any improvement in their life. Freya, for example, lived with multiple physical and mental health conditions compounded by socio-economic disadvantage and extreme social vulnerability. At the time of the first interview, Freya was trying to re-establish her life after she ended a relationship with an abusive partner, saying: "I want to go back to work and do something worthwhile and fulfilling. Being out of work and sick makes me feel worthless and hopeless".

Freya was estranged from most of her family and had few friends. She had lived a transient life, moving frequently and had few social networks in the small rural town to which she had recently relocated. She shares little about her past and physical and mental health conditions with the people in her life saying "I wouldn't say many people know me very intimately". As a result, Freya had few people to draw on in this time of dependency. Being alone was, however, a recurring experience. As she noted: "I've really had to rely on strangers pretty much all throughout my life to get the care that I need and that kind of continues through to this day". Loneliness had been a constant factor in Freya's life, from a childhood of abandonment and trauma, an adolescence lived as an outsider, to an adulthood marked by instability and unpredictability. Being sick and on the margins of society featured heavily in Freya's experience of loneliness and impinged on how she envisioned and planned for her future:

> There's never really been a time where that sense of alienation has really been alleviated, which is why I like activities where I remove myself, in the style of doing things, like plans, because that will give me good release and respite from that profound sense of abandonment. So the loneliness is very closely associated with the sense of abandonment and neglect. (Freya, 40s, with multiple physical and mental health conditions)

At the time of the second interview, Freya's health had declined and she was seeing a neurosurgeon regarding a brain tumour. The intermingled threads of illness, disadvantage, and social and relational factors complicated her ability to manage her health and led her to further social isolation. Faced with insecure housing and financial hardship, Freya was renting a room from a woman with problematic alcohol use who regularly sought Freya's company: "It's a strange situation in that [name of landlady] is lonely and wants someone to talk to but gets herself so drunk and stoned she can't string more than ten words together". Often these bids for connection ended in conflict, which Freya experienced as "uncomfortable, tense and unsafe". Freya longed to move out and create a sense of security and stability for her future but had limited options due to financial constraints and a restricted social network to draw on for assistance. Freya described how her current living situation impacted her mental health, and her ability to trust others:

> Because I am still in extreme hyperarousal—PTSD if you will, and my radar for threats is on red alert. So having someone around with dangerous self-destructive behaviours is not the calming safe home atmosphere I would have hoped for". (Freya, 40s, with multiple physical and mental health conditions)

In discussing the future, Freya hoped to find stable and secure housing and a diagnosis and treatment plan for her tumour. However, she spoke of a future with little hope; a history of life-long and ongoing difficult experiences resulted in despair and exacerbated her feelings of alienation and hopelessness:

> None of this [a stable home and a diagnosis] will stop the painful cycles of endometriosis and the hormonal roller coaster that is severe PMT [premenstrual tension]. I am lonely. I do wish I had someone to listen to me and hold me. I do wish I had someone to be intimate with. I even sucked up my pride and set up a dating profile in the slim hope that there might just be someone out there. But if I'm really honest with myself, I just don't see a romantic connection ever happening again… And the loneliness is just something that I probably just have come to accept, that that's kind of my lot in life. (Freya, 40s, with multiple physical and mental health conditions).

Freya went on to describe how her future was stolen from her due to childhood trauma and illnesses:

> I need to rebuild a core sense of self that can move into my own authenticity, without this miserable grief of my parents hanging over me. I have a right to feel indignation at the complete lack of dignity afforded to me,

> and having my life and future robbed from me by the very people who were supposed to provide a springboard into the world. (Freya, 40s, with multiple physical and mental health conditions)

Freya's future horizon, and her hopes for social connectedness, are thwarted by her illness experiences, past trauma, precariousness and severely constrained resources. For people who experience such existential and biographical uncertainty, planning for the future loses its meaning (Warin et al., 2015).

Conclusion

Chronic illness challenges the normative ordering of time and ideas about progress, productivity and forward motion while jeopardising one's sense of spontaneity and having mastery over one's own time. Thinking with "time" allowed us to draw out how assumptions of linear temporal progression stand in tension with the unfolding, layered and recursive lived experience of chronic conditions. In line with other research on the disruptive and dislocating effects of chronic illness (Bury, 1982), participants' accounts illustrate how the unpredictability of illness unsettled life trajectories, from idealised smooth linearity from past, through present and into the future, to a messy, sometimes chaotic temporal web (Lewis et al., 2022). Furthermore, these accounts highlight the ongoing negotiations of temporalities, materialities, and activities people living with a chronic illness engage in to mitigate loneliness (Cheung et al., 2025).

Exploring chronicity and loneliness through a temporal lens illustrates three main ways chronic illness disrupts experiences of time and how this is related to loneliness. Social norms and ideals are generative of collective rhythms that can be in tension with the personalised rhythms of chronic illness, disrupting a shared world and collective sense of belonging to spaces and places, people and identities for chronically ill people. Although a sense of belonging can lessen loneliness and act as a precursor to social connectedness (Baumeister & Leary, 1995), for people living with chronic illnesses, the disruption to normative temporal markers and horizons fractures the continuity of belonging. Chronic illness brought with it social tensions and discordances arising as participants' lives were lived within the rhythms of managing symptoms, pain and fatigue, while their friends experienced the affective pull of an acceleration of time (Rosa, 2017). Chronic illness introduced aspects into participants' lives that disconnected them from others, from the norm, and from their sense of self. In its absence, a sense of loss and vulnerability arose.

Chronic illnesses limited people's ability to build a sense of belonging across time. Although belonging is unstable and continually claimed and performed, it is also predicated on a degree of "stability, affective concern, and continuation into the foreseeable future" (Baumeister & Leary, 1995, p. 500). Lacking a sense of place in the present, participants struggled to envision a role for themselves in the future. Viewing their future as a foregone conclusion, few narrated the future as representing possibilities for connection and meaning. Chronicity troubled ideals of agentic, autonomous individuals able to chart a certain future. The possibility of a meaningful future was instead understood as something from which they were marginalised. Participants instead conveyed a sense of being stuck in a recursive temporal order, and in a time not of one's own choosing. While May (2017, 2018) has shown that memories of past belonging can be an antidote to present loneliness, these participants' narratives suggest that the relationship between past and present loneliness and belonging is more complicated for those with chronic illness. Chronicity breaks the idea of chronological succession and, in doing so, transforms the (able-bodied) past into a source of anguish and longing. Nostalgia for a previous version of oneself was important in understanding loneliness, as memories of past belonging were a reminder of what had been lost. Participants who traced their loneliness to their diagnosis of chronic illness described loneliness as the gap between their current lived reality and the imagined life they could or should or hoped to have had.

Finally, time for people with chronic illness is differently perceived and experienced, shaped by access to and mobilisation of physical, practical, economic, social, and symbolic resources. The accounts given by Tammy and Freya highlight their sense of stolen futures and their present lack of belonging due to the unpredictability and uncertainty of their illnesses, in relation to disparate financial and social resources. For Tammy, her social and financial security allowed her access to greater resources and supports when she became sick, that were unavailable to Freya. For both women, their experiences of illness shifted their sense of belonging in the world and in the imagined future life course, creating new forms of physical and social precarity in the present. However, without the advantage of social, practical and financial resources to draw on, Freya struggled to establish a sense of belonging and connection to the world. Where Tammy was trying to regain her sense of future, after her illness had limited her ability to build a sense of belonging in time, Freya, in contrast, yearned for a life not lived and held little hope that a different future was possible. These contrasting examples advance our understanding of how social disadvantage contributes to increasing loneliness and ill-health over the life course, demonstrating the inseparability of temporality and materiality.

References

Alacovska, A. (2018). 'Keep hoping, keep going': Towards a hopeful sociology of creative work. *The Sociological Review, 67*(5), 1118–1136. https://doi.org/10.1177/0038026118779014

Baumeister, R., & Leary, M. (1995). The need to belong: Desire for interpersonal attachments as a fundamental human motivation. *Psychological Bulletin, 117*, 497–529. https://doi.org/10.1037/0033-2909.117.3.497

Bury, M. R. (1982). Chronic illness as biographical disruption. *Sociology of Health and Illness, 4*(2), 167–182. https://doi.org/10.1111/1467-9566.ep11339939

Cheung, M. M. Y., Lewis, S., Raja, R., Willis, K., Dubbin, L., Rogers, A., ... & Smith, L. (2025). Disruption and Improvisation: Experiences of Loneliness for People With Chronic Illness. *Qualitative Health Research, 35*(3), 319–334.

Cluley, V., Burton, J. O., Hull, K. L., & Eborall, H. (2024). The paradox of haemodialysis: The lived experience of the clocked treatment of chronic illness. *Health Sociology Review, 33*(1), 24–42.

Harrison, M., Smith, A. K. J., & Adams, S. (2024). Matters of time in health and illness. *Health Sociology Review, 33*(1), 1–9. https://doi.org/10.1080/14461242.2024.2319943

Henning, C. (2017). Thin ties and social context: The importance of meeting places for older persons. *Innovation in Aging, 1*(suppl_1), 1404–1404. https://doi.org/10.1093/geroni/igx004.5169

Hyland, P., Shevlin, M., Cloitre, M., Karatzias, T., Vallières, F., McGinty, G., & Power, J. M. (2019). Quality not quantity: Loneliness subtypes, psychological trauma, and mental health in the US adult population. *Social Psychiatry and Psychiatric Epidemiology, 54*(9), 1089–1099. https://doi.org/10.1007/s00127-018-1597-8

Lewis, S., Willis, K., Franklin, M., & Smith, L. (2022). Challenging times: Disconnects between patient and professional temporalities in chronic condition management. *Critical Public Health, 32*(4), 438–449.

Ljuslinder, K., Ellis, K., & Vikström, L. (2020). Cripping time—understanding the life course through the lens of ableism. *Scandinavian Journal of Disability Research, 22*(1), 35–38. https://doi.org/10.16993/sjdr.710

May, V. (2008). On being a "good" mother: The moral presentation of self in written life stories. *Sociology, 42*(3), 470–486. https://doi.org/10.1177/0038038508088836

May, V. (2018). Belonging across the lifetime: Time and self in mass observation accounts. *The British Journal of Sociology, 69*(2), 306–322. https://doi.org/10.1111/1468-4446.12276

May, V. (2017). Belonging from afar: Nostalgia, time and memory. *The Sociological Review, 65*(2), 401–415.

May, V., & Muir, S. (2015). Everyday belonging and ageing: Place and generational change. *Sociological Research Online, 20*(1), 72–82. https://doi.org/10.5153/sro.3555

Morris, D. (2008). Diabetes, chronic illness and the bodily roots of ecstatic temporality. *Human Studies, 31*(4), 399–421.

Rosa, H. (2017). De-synchronization, dynamic stabilization, dispositional squeeze: The problem of temporal mismatch. In J. Wajcman & N. Dodd (Eds.), *The sociology of speed: Digital, organizational, and social temporalities* (pp. 25–41). Oxford University Press.

Routledge, C., Wildschut, T., Sedikides, C., Juhl, J., & Arndt, J. (2012). The power of the past: Nostalgia as a meaning-making resource. *Memory, 20*(5), 452–460. https://doi.org/10.1080/09658211.2012.677452

Warin, M., Zivkovic, T., Moore, V., Ward, P., & Jones, M. (2015). Short horizons and obesity futures: Disjunctures between public health interventions and everyday temporalities. *Social Science & Medicine*. https://doi.org/10.1016/j.socscimed.2015.01.026

4

Navigating Relationships and Support with Chronic Illness: The Work of Connection

Introduction

Having meaningful relationships with others, including with partners, family members, friends, colleagues and neighbours is important in reducing loneliness and supporting social connectedness across the life-course (Pahl & Spencer, 2004; Rogers et al., 2014; Vela-McConell, 2011). As shown in earlier chapters, the onset of a chronic illness can disrupt valued social relationships and roles, resulting in individuals feeling detached from people in their social networks. However, while supportive relationships are integral to social life, it is claimed (as discussed in Chapter One) that in many societies, the meaningfulness of relationships with others are under challenge due to increasing individualism (Putnam, 2015). Bauman (2012) argues that a defining feature of contemporary societies in neoliberal times is that of "liquid modernity", where forms of modern life are fragile, temporary and vulnerable to constant change; and once solid and enduring social relationships are now uncertain, flexible and "liquid". In such societies, the work of connecting with, and maintaining, one's social relationships has been transformed from a "given" to a "task", meaning that these relationships

S. Lewis et al., *Unravelling the Layers of Chronic Illness and Loneliness*,
https://doi.org/10.1007/978-981-96-7909-6_4

require ongoing renegotiation. The implications for supportive relationships, which is the focus of this chapter, is best captured by Franklin (2009, p. 352), who argues that in liquid modernity:

> ... there is nothing at all to stop those who love you now, who support you now, who employ you now, from dumping you the minute they become bored of you or find a better alternative.

In this chapter, we examine how loneliness and chronic illness intersect to affect interpersonal relationships and experiences of social support, and in turn, how the strength and quality of social bonds within these relationships shapes experiences both with illness and social connectedness. Social bonds comprise the interactions "between social actors as they manifest through alienation, solidarity, attachment and identification with others" (Hurtado Hurtado, 2023 p. 96). Exploring relationships through the lens of social bonds allows us to examine the intricacies of social interactions across different kinds of relationships and how they create, maintain, disrupt and/or reduce social connectedness (Pinquart & Sorensen, 2003), and enable us to make connections between micro-interactions between social actors and larger social ideas, structures and processes (Scheff, 1990, 1997).

Social Relationships: The Social Shaping of Participant Experiences

We asked participants how they navigate social relationships while managing chronic illnesses, who was important to them in feeling more socially connected and how relationships affected their experience of loneliness. Despite extensive variation between the social circumstances of participants in our study, the themes we discuss below about relationships occurred, to varying extents, across all participants. However, some differences in experience emerged when age and household composition were taken into account (Table 1 in Appendix). For those generally younger participants who lived at home, most described supportive family relations. Zarah, Jesinta and May, for example, talked about their mother providing emotional support to them. However, all younger participants (ranging in age from teens to 30s) described struggles with friendships, which contributed to profound feelings of loneliness.

Similarly, although chronic illness put their relationships under strain, participants who lived with their partners, generally (but not always) reported that their partner provided them with support. For example, Elizabeth described her partner as "very supportive", stating "he's been such an important part of not being so hard on myself"; and Tina described her partner as "incredibly empathetic". While Cecilia also described her husband as supportive, she craved affection that was not provided in this relationship. For participants with experiences similar to Elizabeth, Tina and Cecilia, friendships and wider social networks—some long established—are often described as disrupted or strained.

Those participants who lived alone and those with significant caring responsibilities struggled most in attaining and maintaining social bonds, because even limited social support was not available to them at home, or within broader social networks. Jasper and Natalia had caring responsibilities for children, and Phil lived with his mother for whom he was the carer (Chapter Eight also discusses the experience of carers). A few participants talked positively about their neighbours (Bernadette, Bianca and Nick); Ida discussed having a good relationship with her sisters; while a few also talked about positive relationships with healthcare professionals and paid carers. Although Nicola and Michella, who both live alone, have friends, they have not disclosed their illness or their loneliness to them. A common feature of participants who lived alone was that they only identified a very small number of people within their network who provided support. Relationships with animals emerged as important sources of support and connectedness across most participants, though this was most evident in the narratives of people who lived alone. As noted by Franklin (2009), the reliance on more-than-human relationships is a fundamental flow-on effect from social conditions that have resulted in increased loneliness. In light of the different experiences of social bonds, when presenting the themes that emerged from participant accounts, where applicable we also provide information about their living situation.

Shifting Relationships: Imbalances and Misunderstandings

Our analysis of participants' accounts revealed how the presence of illness could strain existing social bonds with partners, family members, friends, and colleagues. Participants reported struggling to connect in meaningful ways with others due to unpredictable symptoms, mental health difficulties, stigmatising experiences and feeling misunderstood. They sought to manage their social relationships in ways that balanced their need for social connectedness with the demands of managing their chronic illness.

Chronic illness introduced imbalances and misunderstandings into relationships, contributing to participants' loneliness. Symptoms like fatigue, pain and nervousness limited what they could do and their capacity to participate in ordinary, routinised ways of socialising with friends and families. These limitations restricted participants' agency over how, when and with whom they interacted. Restricted agency introduced relationship imbalance as many participants felt dependent on the other person to make accommodations and affordances for them. When, as was often the case, other people did not adjust to the participants' new "with-illness" self, the social bond was threatened, as Eloise described:

> I'd lost everything. I'd lost my body, I lost my job, I suddenly realised that because your friends are centred around your hobbies, your sports, your social life, when you can't do that anymore you suddenly discover who your friends really are. And I just knew I couldn't keep up with my friends. …I'm always included in the group message, but no one would ever say, "Eloise, can I come and pick you up?" They still expect me to be the powerful, independent person and it's strange. (Eloise, 60s, with rare neurological autoimmune condition and other chronic conditions)

Participants also described how bonds within existing relationships were threatened when they became "uneven". Feeling unable to fulfil certain expectations that they had of themselves (such as to be a "good" friend or partner) changed the dynamic from one based on reciprocity and interdependency to one of dependency. For Eloise the unevenness of her relationship with her husband provoked feelings of guilt:

> Eloise: At the moment, I don't have a support worker because I really depend a lot on my husband. Because my husband's taken up another job, just financially, we needed some help, so he's gone off and doing some delivery to around the places, just to the door, contactless deliveries. He does a lot of that stuff for me. He workers Saturdays, he has Sundays off. He works Mondays to Saturdays. He's had to take a second job.
> Interviewer: When you say 'had to', for financial reasons?
> Eloise: Financial reasons. Yeah, yeah. Pay for treatment.
> Interview: Yeah okay. So your treatment?
> Eloise: Yeah, yeah. So you can imagine how I feel. Yeah. (Eloise, 60s with rare neurological autoimmune condition and other chronic conditions)

Natalia, a sole parent with two children, described the unevenness that her illness had brought to her relationships, and how this disrupted her sense of how relationships *should* be:

> I should be helping my parents, not them helping me now. I don't want to put that on them. I feel like it actually shouldn't be my friends' and family's responsibility to help me do shopping or help me fix up my garden or put my groceries away for me. I don't feel its right to put things onto other people that really shouldn't be their responsibility. I guess I just don't feel like other people should be responsible for dealing with my disability. (Natalia, 30s, with multiple physical health conditions)

Illustrating how interdependency in relationships could create closeness *and* distance in relationships, Michella, who lives alone, describes how she feared being a burden, being pitied or infantilised by others, while at the same time, recognising that depending on others could also facilitate closeness:

> I have a lot of trouble asking people for help or saying to people, "I'm not doing well." I tend to go to ground and shut everything off, which is doing the opposite of what you should be doing... when somebody does end up coming, afterwards you think, "Oh, that was really nice." I'm always left with good feelings. But I don't think of that in the first place. (Michella, 50s, with systemic lupus erythematosus)

And, as Holly discussed, shrinking social networks also created a fear of becoming "over-reliant" on one or two individuals for social connection and "alienating them":

> When he's [my partner] gone, I was quite sick with that feeling of loneliness. I try not to rely on him. I try to connect with my friends and visit them and talk with them, because I feel that it's really not healthy for me, being the age we are, but it could be any age… I don't want to be left so vulnerable that I'm feeling incapacitated by it, and socially, I don't have any other support network. (Holly, 60s, with urinary incontinence, chronic pain and anxiety)

As discussed in Chapter Two, participants also experienced loneliness in relationships when others misunderstood their illness experience or seemed unable to connect with it. Despite having a positive supportive relationship and knowing that her mother tries to understand, Jesinta illustrates how loneliness can arise from misunderstanding. The ambiguity of her symptoms and how they were understood by both herself and her mother was central to this isolated social bond, and her loneliness:

> Sometimes I'll be sitting down and my mum is sitting across from me and I just feel really alone. Sometimes I'm on the computer talking to my friend and I feel just lonely that they maybe don't quite understand what's going on. Because I have trouble putting everything into words. I think that they're trying to. But I barely even understand what's going on, I can't expect my friends to understand. And I know my mother tries to understand, but she hasn't experienced exactly what's going on. (Jesinta, teens, with autoimmune encephalitis and depression)

In a similar vein, Elizabeth described constantly worrying that people in her network would make erroneous assumptions or judgements about her abilities or character based on their misunderstanding of her condition:

> I don't want people to think that I'm not as capable because I have a health condition. I don't want that to impact. I'm a very driven and

> motivated person and I'm hugely ambitious and I work really hard and I don't want people to think that like, "Oh, is Elizabeth reliable? Can she do that?" And I feel that with my friends even. Like, "Should we book something or is Elizabeth going to get sick?" (Elizabeth, 30s, with chronic bowel obstruction)

Some participants described how close friends or family members appeared uncomfortable discussing their illness and sometimes avoided the topic altogether. Rosemary described the responses from her husband and friends after buying a book about the rehabilitation process for someone who became a quadriplegic, and then subsequently watching the movie (*Penguin Bloom*) with her husband, hoping this would open a conversation about her condition:

> I gave my husband the book to read, and I did tell a few people, and I was sort of hoping that they would say to me, "So, how do you feel? How does this relate to how you feel?" I was hoping that my husband would use that, we could use that to have a bit of a conversation about how I feel. And not one person, not one person has said to me, "So, how does this relate to you?". (Rosemary, 60s, with tick-borne disease and progressive gait disorder)

Similarly, Oliver described the complete avoidance of discussion about his mental health condition, both at home and in his network at church:

> I don't have anyone to be able to talk to about my mental health situation. I have a lot of church friends. But they do not talk about the mental health situation. Even my wife doesn't understand my situation. (Oliver, 50s, with diabetes and schizophrenia)

For participants such as Rosemary and Oliver, avoidance of these discussions contributed to an erasure or diminished visibility of part of their identity, creating distance in their relationship with their partners and friends.

Managing Relationships: Compromises, Trade-Offs and Invisible Work

The physical and emotional work involved in managing and maintaining social relationships while living with chronic illness required participants to make compromises and trade-offs to preserve social connections. Preserving social bonds commanded considerable covert labour, including the work of planning and preparing for a social activity or interaction, managing others' expectations, concealing illness from others and presenting "the best version of themselves". Socialising with chronic illness became a highly staged event rather than a "free-flowing" or spontaneous encounter:

> If I'm going somewhere, I need to plan where I'm going to be. Do I feel comfortable in that environment and how long can I sit there for? I'm not good at going to long shows. I'm better in a restaurant, to see a show than I am in a theatre. I'm no good going to the movies, and overcrowded places are no good for me. (Nick, 50s, with HIV, depression and anxiety disorder)

> Nothing happens organically now. It's not a free-flowing encounter. It feels like it's effort and its stage managed almost and that's not what that's supposed to be. The benefit of being around other people is completely wiped out by the fact that I'm feeling like it's almost a falsehood that takes a great deal of effort to achieve. I'm not really in the moment then. I'm more focused on what I can avoid, rather than what's happening. (Tammy, 40s, with multiple sclerosis (MS))

Moreover, as also discussed in Chapter Three, the work needed to manage chronic illness stole time and energy (already scarce resources) from the labour that was demanded in navigating social relationships. Tina, who reported having a good social network, described the challenges of scheduling a catch-up with a friend around her medical appointments:

> If I don't structure my weeks, I don't see people. And if I put too much energy into prioritising my medical side of things, my health, and I

> pack too much into a week, then where's the time for living? I feel like I go to doctors to continue existing. But life should be more than existing. It should be living, having experience, meeting people, talking to people. So, planning is a big part of that because if I want to see people, I want to hang out, I've got to make sure I've not exhausted myself with medical tests the day before. (Tina, 30s, with multiple physical and mental chronic conditions)

A central challenge for participants was weighing up the desire for social acceptance and belonging against the need to preserve and protect their physical and emotional health and the trade-offs that were required. Bruno (who lives with his parents) and Laura (who lives alone) both articulated how protecting the body and the mind physically and emotionally was often at the expense of social connection (and vice versa):

> My condition limits me to very occasional face-to-face visits, perhaps once a month, with other interaction happening online a little more frequently. My impairments thus make it difficult to develop close relationships with them. This is not just a problem of accessibility; I find social interactions very exhausting, and so while I may have the option to interact with friends more often, these interactions exacerbate my symptoms significantly, so each occasion involves making a decision about whether to make that trade-off. (Bruno, 30s, with chronic fatigue syndrome and anxiety).

> I often have to [cancel plans]. And that can make you lonely as well. Because you want to go. Like I know, I saw the pictures, they would have had a lovely time, but I couldn't go. So then I feel like I'm not connected, because I've missed out on something else. And can I tell any of them the real reason? No. No, no, no, no, no. (Laura, 50s, with arthritis and bipolar disorder)

Bruno went on to describe how his social circle was reduced to a "core group", and he was now careful about which relationships he chose to maintain and give energy to:

> My social life has been curtailed significantly. I have lost contact with most of my old acquaintances and will only visit a core group of friends perhaps once a month. These visits out of the house result in several days of a flu-like worsening of fatigue and depression, but despite this, I consider them to be worth it. (Bruno, 30s, with chronic fatigue syndrome and anxiety)

Others, like Adelaide (living alone in a retirement village), recognised her own precarious social position. Driven by fears of becoming more socially alienated, she fought against her symptoms and the limits of her body to maintain their social relationships and social identities:

> I don't say, "Look, I'm really bloody lonely here." I make sure I keep that connection going so that it won't slip away. And it's only with talking with you this morning that I realised that's what it is, that's what I'm doing, I'm making sure that they don't slip away. (Adelaide, 80s, with pulmonary fibrosis and osteoporosis)

Providing Support in Combating Loneliness

How family members, friends and other social network members supported participants was pivotal in either ameliorating or amplifying their loneliness. Participants felt most supported by those in their networks who treated them as equals and acknowledged and accepted their changing identity by validating their illness experience. For some participants like Ida, this meant forging new friendships or partnerships:

> I still do feel embarrassed. But I've been out a couple times with him [my partner] and he doesn't seem to worry. He can see that I can't walk very well and I bang into things. If we go somewhere and I have to go to the loo, well, he's got to help me to the door of the toilet because I can't walk on my own. So, he seems okay with that, yeah, which is good. It was nice to go out somewhere as an adult, an adult with another adult. (Ida, 60s, with MS)

Some participants commented that they felt supported when others adjusted how they interacted together or their expectations of the relationship. For Bruno, having friends who were able to bend and mould to the unpredictability and changing demands of his illness supported him in maintaining connections:

> I have lost touch with many friends I knew from around the time I fell ill. But I consider myself very fortunate to still have an (albeit small) group of friends, not just because they are good people, but because the settings in which I visit with them are reasonably accommodating and relaxed affairs. (Bruno, 30s, with chronic fatigue syndrome and anxiety)

As Bruno describes (above), however, it depended on the other person making accommodations. He added that:

> Because I am only able to visit friends when my symptoms are least severe, they do not witness the exacerbation of symptoms that occurs in the days afterwards, they are unlikely to know the full extent of my impairment. [Thus] the support I get from friends is mostly indirect. (Bruno, 30s, with chronic fatigue syndrome and anxiety)

Participants commented that in most of their relationships, due to hidden or misunderstood symptoms, the other party did not make accommodations to how or where they socialised.

Very few participants described forging connections with individuals or communities based on similar experiences of illness (Laura and Betty's experience of an online support is discussed in Chapter Six). Bruno attributed this both to how chronic illness forces social withdrawal as well as the invisibility of symptoms:

> I do not personally know anyone that shares my illness, which I partially attribute to the fact that they would be similarly socially withdrawn for the same reasons I am. The term 'invisible illness' takes on an additional meaning because of this. (Bruno, 30s, with chronic fatigue syndrome and anxiety)

Others like Eloise, who lives with a rare neurological condition that primarily affects older people, had sought support from an illness-related peer support group, but she did not return as she shared nothing in common (outside of the diagnosis) with the other group members.

Feeling seen by others was also important in ameliorating loneliness (explored in-depth in Chapter Two). Friends and family who were able to strike a balance between validating their illness experience (e.g. not minimising it or pretending the illness did not exist) and recognising them for their whole personhood—that is, as "more than" their illness identity, facilitated a sense of connection and reciprocity in the relationship. Tammy described how supported she feels with friends who see, accept, and validate the "multiple layers" of her personhood:

> I think that people who are genuinely good friends, good social connections, they see past it or they acknowledge it and they just see it as being part of who you are [whereas] some people are so aware of it that they're hypersensitive. I want to be the person that I was before with them and have all the other layers of who I am and let them feel comfortable and secure enough to talk to me about what's going on with them too. Because that's what a two-sided friendship is to me. (Tammy, 40s, with MS)

Many participants discussed the importance of feeling seen and valued by those who they did not know well, including casual encounters with café and supermarket staff, or people that they saw in their neighbourhoods, as well as across on- and off-line spaces. For participants like Nicola, these "small conversations" with people in her local neighbourhoods helped her feel less alone and more connected to her community, despite having few or no close social connections. Nicola's quote below illustrates the powerful effects of casual encounters, particularly for people who live alone. As she described, the seemingly small act of recognition (the barista knowing her coffee order), could be a powerful force in connecting people to their community:

> For me they're [casual encounters] important, because otherwise I'm completely by myself. To be able to have a face-to-face physical conversation is quite grounding, in a way, because you're in that moment and

> it's not a screen. There is one cafe that I have frequented quite a bit. The barista is fantastic. He's one of those people where you walk in and he serves you coffee and he's like, "Here," and you just have a small conversation or a short conversation and that's that. So, I do have that. I think it's nice that someone knows my coffee order. (Nicola, 30s, with MS)

Friends and family could also provide the wrong kind of support. Even if well-intended, some interactions intensified participants' loneliness. Participants described unhelpful supports such as what they perceived to be "hollow" or superficial expressions of sympathy or pity, attempts by others to shield the participant from potential social threats or stigmatising encounters, attempts by others to "fix" the problem by "forcing" social engagement onto them, or offering unsolicited advice (such as to join a group, volunteer, or attend an event):

> I've literally had to say to family and friends, "Don't come. I don't want you to come." And my mother even did turn up one day and I felt like, "This is exhausting." I just had to be as nice as I could, but I wasn't. It was a struggle. (Tammy, 40s, with MS)

> They don't understand. Nobody obviously understands, because they're not walking in your shoes sort of thing, but they do understand your limitations. They understand that it's depressing and that. But they just tell me to buck up and, "Come on, get in, we're going," sort of thing. When I get a bit down or anything, and I don't really want to go anywhere, they just say, "Oh come on" and you've got to go sort of thing. (Ida, 60s, with MS)

What unified these supports described as "unhelpful" was a clear disconnect between the support the participant wanted to help them feel more connected and what the other party believed was helpful. This is illustrated below by Betty (who lives alone) talking about her partner. While she wanted to share her experience of loneliness with her partner, she did not feel comfortable doing this, fearing that her partner would attempt to "fix the problem" rather than simply listen to and understand her. This misunderstanding between Betty and her partner minimised her lived experience of loneliness and chronic illness, making her feel even more alone:

> Last night after the interview I really wanted to share it with somebody, and I really wanted it to be him. So, I don't think it's so much a fear of loneliness as a desire for connection... Because he's a fixer, and I don't need anybody to fix me. I'm busy doing it myself. Go fix yourself and then we'll talk. See, he's always trained to extract the thing that needs to be fixed, and then tell me how to fix it. It's a bit uncomfortable. (Betty, 40s, with chronic pain, musculoskeletal issues and post-traumatic stress disorder (PTSD))

Non-Human Companionship

As we have shown above, a prominent feature across participants' accounts was that their social bonds with people in their networks are complicated, fragile, insecure and contingent on the undulations of chronic illness. The fragility, tenuousness, and need of performativity evident in participants interpersonal relationships, has according to Franklin (2009) been one of the drivers behind the dramatic growth in companion pets, referring to the "crisis of intimacy, love and companionship in Western societies" (p. 350). In the absence of meaningful relationships with other people, participants talked at length in their interviews about both companion and non-companion animals as vital sources of companionship, comfort, love and support. This was evident in the effusive language that participants used to describe their companion animals and the bond that they shared with them: "she is a source of joy", "I so love her", "I adore her" and "he is the most precious thing in the world to me". Participants' animals also featured in the photographs shared during photo elicitation and walking interviews, as can be seen in photographs from Verna, Michella, Rosemary, and Jessica (Images 4.1, 4.2, 4.3, 4.4).

As is evident below, the bond that Luke (who lives alone) and Jesinta (who lives with her parents and siblings) have with their companion animals offers a protective and supportive presence and comfort when they are feeling lonely, sad or afraid:

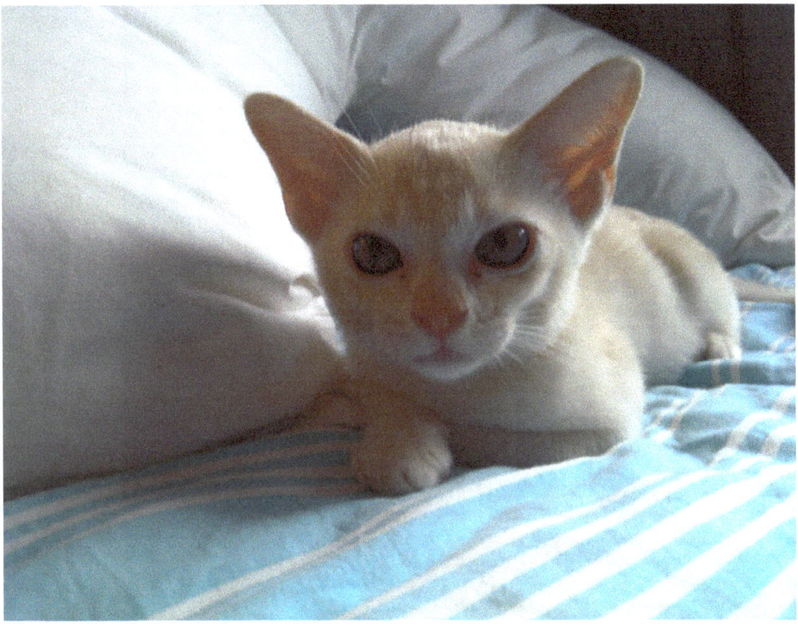

Image 4.1 Verna's photograph of one of her cats described as something to love and be loved by

> She's a smoocher, this one. But I love it. If it wasn't for her, I wouldn't use my larynx in the morning. Because as soon as she hears my bed, I have a high low bed, as soon as I lower it, she hears it, she gets off her bed, come over and she licks my hand so I know where she is and I'll say, "Good morning, Bella. How are you little girl? Hey, where's my little girl." And you don't know what that does for me. Oh, and I love her. She, I guess, helps me to get over that, being lonesome. Because you can pet her, talk to her, and she does respond. (Luke, 60s, with visual impairment, chronic pain and other chronic conditions)

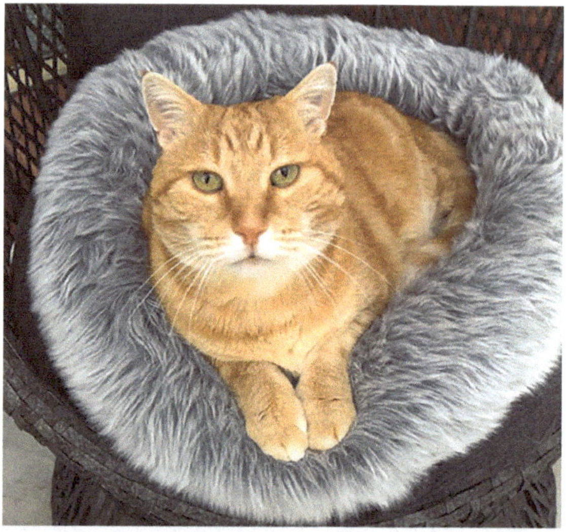

Image 4.2 Michella's photograph of her cat, keeping her company at home

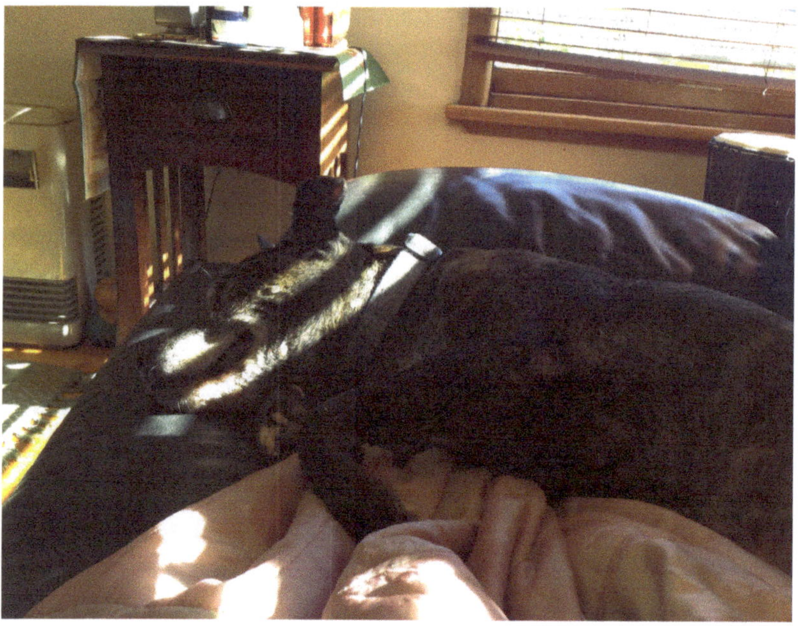

Image 4.3 Rosemary's photograph of her dog, her daily companion in the home and on walks

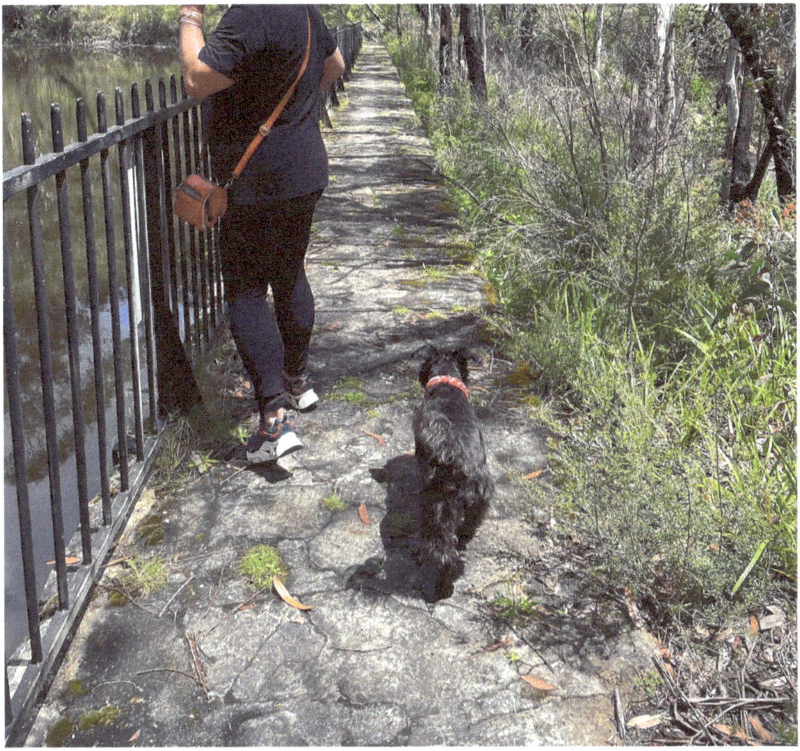

Image 4.4 Jessica's dog, taken on her walking interview in the bush

I've got two cats. One's right there and one's right over there. They're both with me. They're so important to me. I used to hide in the closet when I was sad or scared, and they would always try and open the closet door and sit in with me. They didn't like me crying. I think they think it was sad. So, right now, I'm alone in this room so they're both here watching over me. Nigel is standing guard by the door and Rogue is sitting right next to me on the floor. And I see that as standing guard for me and protecting me. It's just the best when you're feeling nauseous or you've got a bad headache or you're crying because you've gained weight again, all these things. You can just come to your cat and just be like, "Rogue, I'm sad," and she'll purr and give you a lick and give you kisses and boop you. (Jesinta, teens, with autoimmune encephalitis, and depression)

Relationships with companion animals were also valued because they offered the person a sense of social value and self-worth, as they enabled them to care for and care about another being, in a way that was often denied to them by others in their networks (e.g. when they were rendered the care recipient or the dependent in the relationship). For Elizabeth, being able to care and be dependable helped her "come back out of myself":

> Having my pets has been life-changing... not being home alone or having someone at home, just totally changed, and being responsible for somebody else. That was a significant turning point I think, getting my rabbit, because I think it has helped me to come back out of myself. I had to be there with it and I had to be present and I had to feed her and I had to—I'm always in routine. I forced myself to stay in my routine to keep going. And I think getting a pet was a huge, huge life change. Yeah, that was actually probably the biggest shift when I got Daisy, and then just spending time with her in the afternoon. I know she's an animal, but socialising with anything, as opposed to just coming home to nothing, and sitting at home. (Elizabeth, 30s, with chronic bowel obstruction)

Some participants like Cecilia, below, recounted that her husband bought her a dog to provide companionship as she transitioned to a more sedentary life due to her illness:

> I've got this gorgeous toy poodle. She is just a gem. She loves to get on my lap. And as soon as she sees me put the chair up and get the blanket on the lap, she's on my lap as quick as lightning. (Cecilia, 70s, with complications after a lung transplant)

For others, their dogs helped draw them into the fold of community life. Walking in dog parks and enjoying interactions with other people's dogs was also described as a strategy to reduce loneliness. While connecting with a dog was important in itself, these interactions also served as a safe and easy topic to spark incidental conversations with other humans, as Nelly, who lives alone with her cat, regularly visits the local dog park, discusses:

> I find animals easier to talk to maybe. I don't know. And people always want to talk about their animals. (Nelly, 70s, with chronic obstructive pulmonary disease (COPD)).

While Nelly talked about how dogs helped her connect with other people, Greg in a similar vein, described how having a dog brought other people into his world:

> When you're in a carpark and you're there all day, you get to talk to a lot of people. And if you've got a dog, you get to talk to even more, because everyone wants to pat him. "Oh, can I throw the stick for him?" "Oh, what a lovely dog," so conversations start up. (Greg, 60s, with chronic back pain)

Although not a companion animal in the conventional sense, Nelly also discussed, with joy, "my possum"—a native animal that now lives in one of her hanging garden baskets:

> I've got a possum. It's lovely. I have possums all around the house and I don't ever see them near. They come out at night and they play in my garden and leave poo everywhere and then they take off. But the other day I was watering, and I watered this hanging basket and out jumped this possum with a baby on her back. I ran inside and I locked my cat in, because my cat would have a go at it I'm sure. And she was up on a rafter and I waited a half an hour, and in that half an hour she disappeared, so I thought, "Fine." Lo and behold the next day she's back in the pot plant again, in the hanging basket. So, she decided she's going to live in there. So now I don't water this plant. I'm going to lose this plant because I don't want to water it because of my possum (Nelly, 70s, with COPD).

Conclusion

Despite one of the most often cited definitions of loneliness being that it manifests as deficit between desired and actual social relationships, much of the scholarship about loneliness uncritically posits social relationships as inherently beneficial in protecting against loneliness. Our analysis reveals a more complicated picture of how multiple relationships and their dynamic social bonds are associated with loneliness, specifically how relational dynamics and interactions can simultaneously foster intimacy and support, as well as conflict and distance. The lens of social bonds is helpful in examining how relationships and their dynamics change in relation to the undulations, unpredictability and multiplicity of illness. The complexities of relationships in participants' daily lives reveal how chronic illness renders social bonds precarious, how relationships with different individuals can either help or harm efforts to address loneliness, and how different kinds of loneliness—emotional and social—manifest within and across these different relationships.

As we have seen in this chapter, social bonds are tenuous for many participants with chronic illness, and they struggle with misunderstandings, invalidations, conflict, reciprocity, and dependency—all of which can place their relationships under strain (Blatterer, 2015). The personal struggles these individuals experienced cannot be separated from our broader social context, particularly the high cultural currency placed on individualism (discussed in Chapter One). Bauman (2012) argues in *Liquid Modernity* that relationships in a society that privileges individualism undermine the stability of social bonds:

> A most salient aspect of the vanishing act performed by old securities is the new fragility of human bonds. The brittleness and transience of bonds may be an unavoidable price for individuals' *right* to pursue their individual goals (Bauman, 2012, p. 170).

This individualistic ethos directly shaped how participants navigated social relationships with chronic illness. Many described a slow decline in meaningful and authentic connections over time, associated with their fear of being "too dependent" or "too needy". The social norms that elevate independence, while stigmatising vulnerability and dependency, are implicated in their experience of loneliness (Brooks et al., 2020; Peacock et al., 2019). For participants, this created a painful paradox: their chronic conditions necessitated greater reliance on others, yet their fear of violating these deeply ingrained social values led them to withdraw, ultimately amplifying their experience of loneliness.

As we discussed in Chapter Two, how chronic illness is seen or unseen, interpreted or misinterpreted, and responded to within interpersonal relationships, can place social bonds under strain and contribute to loneliness. While some research shows that people with illness value connections forged with peers or fellow sufferers (Lewis et al., 2024), in our study most participants had not formed these kinds of bonds. Finding or gaining access to individuals and communities with shared illness experiences was extremely difficult due to factors such as the invisibility of symptoms and the complexities of living with multiple chronic physical and mental illnesses.

The social rules governing different kinds of relationships can be in competition or tension with the demands of managing the illness. Socially prescribed ways of "showing up" in relationships can collide with need for self-care and recovery, upsetting the dynamics of the relationship and its reciprocity. Relationships in which social bonds are flexible—that is, they bend to the undulations of the illness and accommodate (and even embrace) new with-illness identities—can protect against loneliness and are highly valued. The more commonly described experience was that of inflexibility in relationships that rendered the person with chronic illness feeling the need to undertake significant emotional work in maintaining the relationship, as well as sometimes sacrifice self-care and endure pain or fight against their body (Moensted et al., 2023; Spencer et al., 2021).

Participants also described a mismatch between the support they needed to mitigate feelings of loneliness and the support that was provided. The emotional work associated with supporting someone with chronic illness includes the provision of comfort and support, validating and supporting reassessments of identity and the future, and understanding and responding to the multiple dimensions of chronic illness (Vassilev et al., 2013). Yet in many cases, while relationships described by participants provided practical support, such as assistance in daily living, managing medical appointments, and well-intentioned actions like encouraging social outings and activities, it was the emotional work of chronic illness in social bonds (and in many cases the absence of this) that had most impact on loneliness. The importance of bonds with non-human animals in ameliorating feelings of loneliness for participants illustrates the critical importance of approaches to loneliness that go beyond a focus on cultivating meaningful connection with other humans. Unlike human relationships, which were often governed by expectations of reciprocity and performance, relationships with other animals offered acceptance and non-judgemental companionship, without the requirement to disclose illness experience, the labour of managing relationships during periods of illness intensification, or the potential for social rejection. This finding highlights the importance of more expansive approaches to loneliness that recognise that social bonds extend beyond interpersonal relationships, to encompass a broader range of connections through which people find belonging.

References

Bauman, Z. (2012). *Liquid Modernity*. Polity Press, Cambridge (original date of publication 2000).

Blatterer, H. (2015). *Everyday friendships: Intimacy as freedom in a complex world*. Palgrave Macmillan UK.

Brooks, H. L., Bee, P., Lovell, K., & Rogers, A. (2020). Negotiating support from relationships and resources: A longitudinal study examining the role of personal support networks in the management of severe and enduring mental health problems. *BMC Psychiatry, 20*(1), 50. https://doi.org/10.1186/s12888-020-2458-z

Franklin, A. S. (2009). On loneliness. *Geografiska Annaler: Series B, Human Geography, 91*(4), 343–354. https://doi.org/10.1111/j.1468-0467.2009.00326.x

Hurtado Hurtado, J. (2023). Towards a postmortal society of virtualised ancestors? The virtual deceased person and the preservation of the social bond. *Mortality, 28*, 1–16.

Lewis, S., Newton, G., Kenny, K., & Boyle, F. (2024). The incurable self: Negotiating social bonds and dis/connection with metastatic breast cancer. *Sociology of Health & Illness, 46*(2), 295–314.

Moensted, M. L., Lewis, S., Willis, K., Dubbin, L., Rogers, A., & Smith, L. (2023). Friendship, connectedness and (in)authenticity for those with chronic illness: Trading in one social gain for another. *SSM-Qualitative Research in Health, 3*, Article 100246. https://doi.org/10.1016/j.ssmqr.2023.100246

Pahl, R., & Spencer, L. (2004). Personal communities: Not simply families of 'fate' or 'choice.' *Current Sociology, 52*(2), 199–221. https://doi.org/10.1177/0011392104041808

Peacock, M., Bissell, P., & Owen, J. (2019). Dependency denied: Health inequalities in the neo-liberal era. *Social Science & Medicine, 118*, 173–180.

Pinquart, M., & Sorensen, S. (2003). Risk factors for loneliness in adulthood and old age—a meta-analysis. In S. P. Shohov (Ed.), *Advances in Psychology Research* (vol. 19, pp. 111–143). Nova Science

Putnam, R. D. (2015). Bowling alone: America's declining social capital. In *The city reader* (pp. 188–196). Routledge

Rogers, A., Brooks, H., Vassilev, I., Kennedy, A., Blickem, C., & Reeves, D. (2014). Why less may be more: A mixed methods study of the work and relatedness of 'weak ties' in supporting long-term condition self-management. *Implementation Science, 9*(1), 19. https://doi.org/10.1186/1748-5908-9-19

Scheff, T. J. (1990). Microsociology: Discourse, emotion, and social structure. University of Chicago Press, Chicago.

Scheff, T. J. (1997). Emotions, the social bond, and human reality: Part/whole analysis. Cambridge University Press, Cambridge.

Spencer, G., Lewis, S., & Reid, M. (2021). The agentic self and uncontrollable body: Young people's management of chronic illness at university. *Health, 25*(3), 357–375.

Vassilev, I., Rogers, A., Blickem, C., Brooks, H., Kapadia, D., Kennedy, A., & Reeves, D. (2013). Social networks, the 'work' and work force of chronic illness self-management: A survey analysis of personal communities. *PLoS ONE, 8*(4), Article e59723. https://doi.org/10.1371/journal.pone.0059723

Vela-McConnell, J. (2011). *Unlikely friends bridging ties and diverse friendships.* Lexington Books.

5

Reaching in, Branching out: Strategies for Navigating Loneliness

Introduction

In previous chapters we have focused on how loneliness is experienced and understood personally, within family and friendship groups, and in relation to illness trajectories and life course. Loneliness adds another undesirable psychosocial layer of complexity to life with illness. For people with chronic conditions loneliness becomes an additional dimension to be managed. As discussed in Chapter One, loneliness when viewed as an individual issue is something individuals *should* be able to "fix", through individual actions, prescribed self-management behaviours or "good" lifestyle choices (Sagan & Jones, 2024). Neves et al. (2019) when researching loneliness in aged care, found that alleviation of loneliness was seen as individual responsibility, even when structural causes of loneliness were recognised. In light of these dominant cultural ideas about loneliness and individual responsibility, understanding how people with chronic conditions address their loneliness is important—in particular, the opportunities they feel to exercise agency over their situation and the barriers they experience in doing so.

S. Lewis et al., *Unravelling the Layers of Chronic Illness and Loneliness*, https://doi.org/10.1007/978-981-96-7909-6_5

Previous research has focused mostly on how older and younger adults attempt to overcome loneliness, pointing out that variations in the experience of loneliness over time, both in its intensity and in its persistence, require people who experience loneliness to draw on multiple strategies (Kharicha et al., 2021). The need to shift one's mindset using cognitive strategies or engaging in other activities has been identified (Kharicha, 2021; Verity et al., 2021; Neves et al., 2019). Specifically, young people talk about the need for "distraction" strategies and creating positive moments (Verity et al., 2021); older adults identify the need for cognitive strategies that enable them to reframe their negative feelings (Kharicha et al., 2021), or distraction through "doing something" (Neves et al., 2019). Across both these populations there is the need for supportive relationships, with research indicating that while sometimes lonely individuals need to be proactive in engaging with others, responsibility also lies with peers and other professionals (such as teachers for young people) to recognise and respond to indicators of loneliness (Verity et al., 2021).

In research with older people experiencing loneliness, Kharicha et al. (2021) differentiated between strategies that were implemented in an "inside world" and an "outside world". Inside world strategies were generally kept private from others and focused on managing one's negative feelings in an attempt to "make the feelings more manageable" (Kharicha et al., 2021, p. 1207). "Outside world" strategies focused on engagement and connections with others (see also Neves et al., 2019). These strategies included engagement with place through spending time outdoors, and purposively seeking out meaningful interactions or activities with others, all of which required considerable effort. A review by Shi et al. (2023) noted that chronic conditions impact the capacity to engage in both inside and outside worlds. As discussed in Chapter Two, onset of a chronic illness can disrupt one's sense of self and biography; and strategies to overcome loneliness may also be directed towards repairing or restoring lost self-identify (Bury, 1991; Charmaz, 1994). Shi et al. (2023) found that while socialising with others is integral to addressing loneliness, "self-strategies" were also needed to address both loneliness and chronic conditions. These self-strategies include reconstructing self-identities, rethinking biographies, and staying occupied.

For people with chronic illnesses, managing one's identity and the expectations of others is inextricably entangled with the experience of loneliness, as discussed in earlier chapters. Goffman's (1959) dramaturgical work on impression management provides a framework for understanding how and why individuals seek to manage how others view them; for example, through managing the setting in which they are likely to be viewed (and judged) by others. For Goffman, face-to-face social interactions occur on a "frontstage", where interactions can be shaped to present the self, as well as the accompanying expectations of participants in social interactions. On the other hand, the "backstage" is the site where individuals can put aside their performance in the knowledge that no viewers are judging their performance. For people with chronic illnesses, the backstage can provide much-needed respite from frontstage, particularly when symptoms are variable or unpredictable. However, changes in how we engage socially, such as increased use of digital communications may disrupt the separation of these two spheres of impression management. Some have argued that there is now a blurring of boundaries between backstage and frontstage (Beames et al., 2021). As we discuss further in Chapter Six, one implication of the growth in online communication, especially social media, is the pervasiveness of presenting oneself continually—always being "on". People with chronic illnesses therefore manage themselves, their illness, and their interactions in these digital spaces without the benefits afforded by the private (backstage) work needed to maintain their frontstage identity.

In this chapter, we discuss the strategies that people who are lonely and living with chronic illnesses described implementing to address their loneliness, showing how the strategies they deploy are often framed within a social and cultural milieu that emphasises individual responsibility and treats loneliness as undesirable. Thus, in participant accounts, there is a focus on individual actions, rather than a focus on broader socially constituted strategies that change the environment within which loneliness occurs. Loneliness was seen as an 'I' problem, rather than a 'we' or 'us' problem; and the language of individual responsibility permeated participants' accounts.

One participant, Elizabeth, explains how the undesirability of loneliness and the focus on individual responsibility is experienced. Elizabeth, in her early thirties, has lived with chronic bowel issues since childhood.

Living alone and often hospitalised, she described battling with severe depression and episodes of loneliness. Despite having friends who also experience chronic illness, she found disclosing her loneliness particularly difficult due to the stigma associated with being lonely:

> I think that also comes down to that perception that is driven often by the perception that you shouldn't be lonely. You should be able to deal with that. You shouldn't feel that way. You should be fine by yourself. (Elizabeth, 30s, with chronic bowel obstruction)

Internal to the Mind: Distraction, Positive Thinking and "Self-Discipline"

Embracing the idea of self-responsibility to address loneliness, participants in our study described working hard to change their negative experiences of loneliness. Participants overwhelmingly discussed the need to change their feelings by thinking, feeling or acting differently. Michella, in her fifties, experienced daily pain and fatigue from her autoimmune condition. She described focusing on "zoning out" "to stop stressing about things or to stop dwelling on being lonely or sad". Almost all participants talked about the need to "distract" themselves from the unpleasant feelings of loneliness with strategies conducted in solitude (see also Cheung et al., 2024). Renee talked about the emotional dimensions of loneliness and struggled to articulate any strategy beyond distraction that worked to alleviate this:

> If I start getting worried and frightened and down, I'll try and distract myself with something. That's probably about the only strategy. (Renee, 70s, with chronic obstructive pulmonary disease (COPD))

Many participants talked about reading, watching television, or listening to music as important distraction strategies. Nicola described watching "comedies or light-hearted fun stuff" to "lift loneliness a bit". She focused on undertaking small manageable activities every day that could ward off unpleasant feelings:

> I try and do something nice for myself every day, so that generally is get a coffee or whatever. They're not massive things. Well, it's about distraction really. That's all this is. A distraction from the shitty things (Nicola, 30s, with multiple sclerosis (MS))

Similarly, Eloise and Oliver described strategies that provided distraction and were conducted in solitude:

> I try and paint. So again, it's in isolation. Paint, music, reading, take the dog for a little walk. (Eloise, 60s, with rare neurological autoimmune condition and other chronic conditions)

> When I cannot go to sleep usually, during that lonely situation, I turn onto my music. (Oliver, 50s, with diabetes and schizophrenia)

When Eloise was no longer able to go outside to paint in nature due to her pain, she turned one of the rooms in her house into her painting room. She shared a collage of photographs that contrasted her pre-illness life painting in nature with friends, with-illness life painting at home from her memories. As she articulates in her caption, while painting in solitude was calming, it was also lonely (Image 5.1).

Participants also utilised the Internet to ward off loneliness. Adelaide described spending hours, daily, doing Internet-based research related to her hobbies such as astrology, psychology, and history. Toby and Zarah were both often homebound due to fatigue. Toby described videogaming to "block out" loneliness:

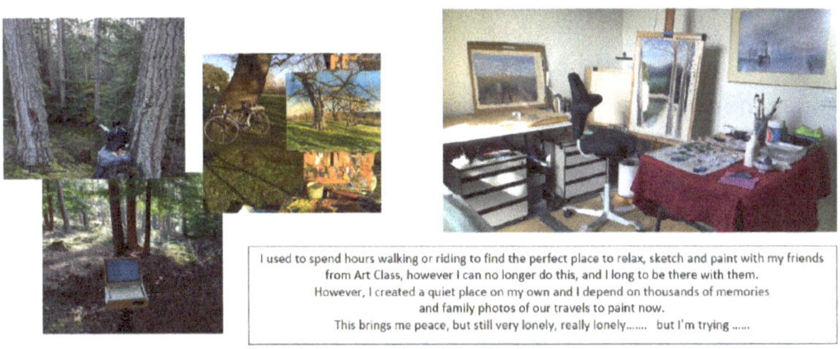

Image 5.1 Eloise's photographs of painting before and after illness

> I try and get something in the way of it, something that blocks it out, just doing something else that would stop me from feeling that [loneliness]. Something where you don't have to think about that. I don't know. Something that when you would focus, would not do it. Because I feel your focus would be pulled by the loneliness again… I don't know, just playing video games or something. (Toby, 20s, with rare genetic condition causing weakness, fatigue and concentration difficulties)

Zarah used social media as a way to "numb" herself:

> I'll go on social media or something and just try and forget. It kind of just numbs. It doesn't solve it, but it just makes you forget it. I might have some sort of snack or eat something. Some emotional eating or something. But yeah, there's not much to do. I just try and distract myself. (Zarah, 20s, with MS and depression)

Participants also discussed how planning activities with a view to "keeping busy" kept feelings of loneliness at bay. As Adelaide said: "I've made the effort to include activities in my life to prevent that [loneliness] and make me busy". Ida, a retired clerical worker in her early 60s who, due to MS and neuralgia, was largely homebound described loneliness as associated with boredom and feeling "trapped" inside: "You feel lonely in the house. Sometimes you just think, 'I've got to get out of this house.'" Ida described how the knowledge that she had activities planned for the week that would get her out of the house lessened her loneliness. Planning pleasurable activities was itself a distraction strategy:

> But when you've got something to look forward to its good. When you're going to have a day at home you've got to think, "Now, what am I going to do tomorrow?" You have to give yourself something to do, like a task. (Ida, 60s, with MS)

Similarly, as shown in Images 5.2 and 5.3, Betty had an array of self-care strategies that focused her attention to the activities that she needed to do and take stock if she had large gaps in the week where she felt alone or had nothing to do. In talking about the significance of Image 5.2 she said:

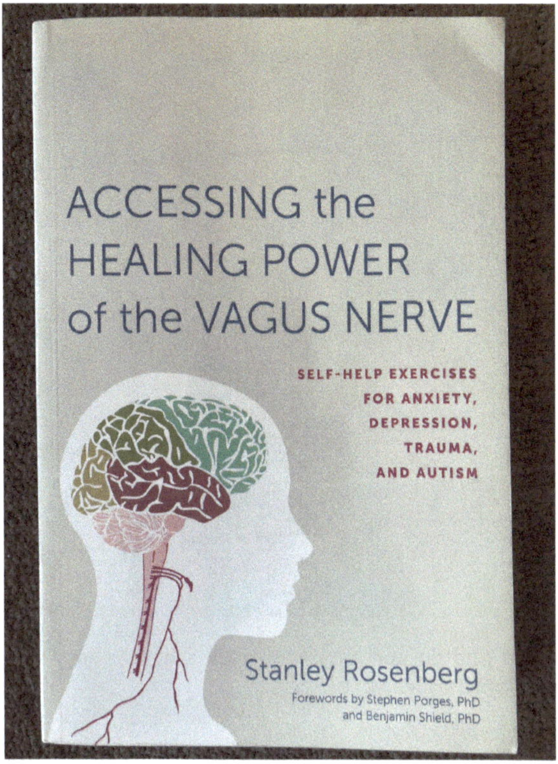

Image 5.2 Betty's photograph of a book she reads regularly as part of her self-care strategy

> ...if I want to get better I need to regulate and retrain my nervous system so that I'm in rest and digest or a certain engagement consistently. And so, that book is one of the learning tools I've been using to try and heal. (Betty, 40s, with chronic pain, musculoskeletal issues, and post-traumatic stress disorder (PTSD))

The personal strategy of distracting oneself to ameliorate loneliness was entwined with social perceptions. Participants described distraction strategies in the context of the social undesirability of dependence on others ("not wanting to be a burden on others") and the fear of rejection if they disclosed their lonely feelings to others. The struggles and

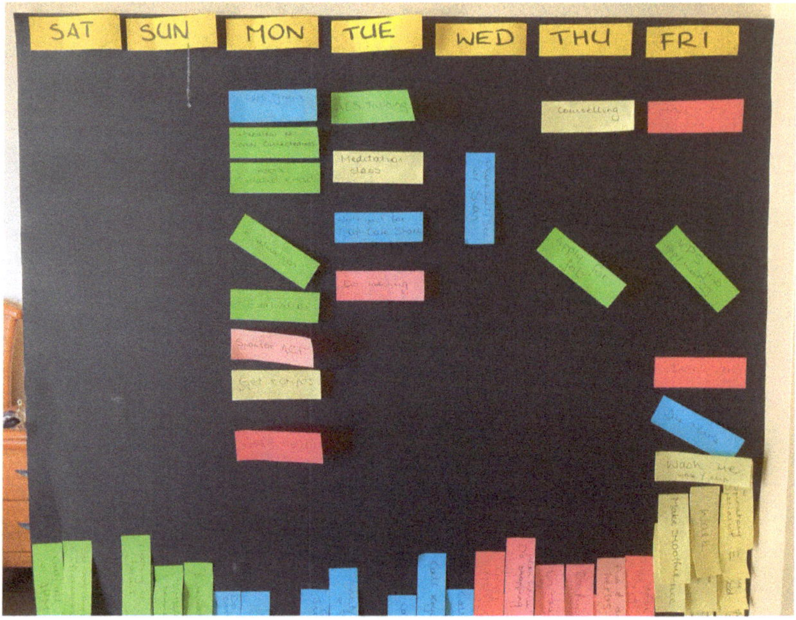

Image 5.3 Betty's photograph of her weekly schedule which she created to keep busy and prioritise social activities

the limits of distraction are described by Bianca, in her early sixties. Due to multiple health conditions, including autoimmune conditions, Bianca was limited in the types of activities she could attend. Bianca described previously being part of a larger community which had slowly dwindled as her ability to participate in this community decreased. Although the loss of community had isolated her, she was reluctant to disclose her feelings to others. She focused on distraction strategies rather than burdening or relying on others for help:

> It has helped me over the years to focus on a project or focus on an idea. Because even at night sometimes I'm sitting here and thinking, "Oh, I want to talk to someone." And I think, "Oh, I don't want to bother them." I say, "Well, what can I do to get myself out of here? I'm in a horrible spot, I'm feeling isolated, I'm feeling disconnected, and all of that." So, I often think, "I need to get myself out." And, of course,

> writing, getting in my head, focusing. And that's when I said, "I've got to get back into what helps me if I can't rely on people to help me, or I can't go out and enjoy a walk on the beach to rejuvenate me." ...So now, I've gotten into this book and I'm doing the research and doing the planning for it, I'm thinking of conversations. So, my mind is extracted away from my own issues. (Bianca, 60s, with fibromyalgia and severe food and chemical sensitivities)

Cognitive strategies extending beyond distraction were also discussed by participants. Some described reframing by reflecting on their place in the world and emphasising a strong mindset. Situating one's emotions within a broader context, social comparison and thinking positively helped these participants gain perspective about their feelings. As Phil and Elizabeth described:

> I always look on the positive. If something goes wrong, I go and check how 90% of the population is doing so much worse than I am. (Phil, 60s, with osteoporosis and schizophrenia)

> Instead of focusing on the sadder feelings just find the light. It would be very easy to find the darkest, but instead I just try and focus on what's positive. I actively work to find those positives and to find the light so that I don't dwell too much on those darker times per se. (Elizabeth, 30s, with chronic bowel obstruction)

Similarly, Rory discussed the need for both distraction and mindfulness strategies; but acknowledged that these strategies only offered partial amelioration of loneliness. Rory is a non-binary person in their late fifties. They moved to a rural area two years ago with their then-wife, although they divorced shortly after. At the time of the interview, Rory was feeling the impact of moving to a new town and having to re-establish friendships and connections. Despite having made two friends in the town, Rory missed having family and close friends around, particularly the type of "taken-for-granted but close" connections they had growing up. Rory had a severe work-related accident 20 years ago which led to chronic back problems, prolapsed discs, sciatica pain and fibromyalgia. Being unable to work since the accident, Rory developed depression, anxiety, and social anxiety, which they felt complicated the establishment of new friendships. Rory discussed their strategies to manage loneliness such as distraction and mindfulness exercises:

> I try and distract myself from it usually, in one way or another. Try and bring other thoughts to mind, do something just actively, go for a walk, play with my dogs that I've got, put the television on, put the radio on, listen to some music. Sometimes, rather than distracting myself, I might deal with it in a positive way by doing, say, mindfulness exercises. Just bringing in the world around me and acknowledging it and acknowledging where I am and how I'm feeling. (Rory, 50s, with fibromyalgia, chronic pain, and depression)

However, distraction and mindfulness have their limits. Rory often felt lonely, missed being part of a community, and especially missed having "mid-level friends"—that is, people who were more than acquaintances—which would allow them to draw less on their two main friends. Having more friends would also make Rory feel more socially accepted and integrated into the rural community. Rory discussed how social vulnerability founded in a limited network made disclosing loneliness feel additionally risky:

> Often there can be an element of risk taking. That you dare share something vulnerable or difficult, risking, from your past experience, that people can turn you away when you say that you're having troubles. (Rory, 50s, with fibromyalgia, chronic pain, and depression)

Focusing inwards affords self-protection in the face of possible rejection when you are not able to present the best version of yourself to others. Later in the interview, Rory talked about the constraints of sharing—the risks of exposing one's vulnerability and also not wanting to burden others:

> People are often uncomfortable with vulnerability and with others demonstrating or talking about their vulnerability. And that can be quite off-putting for other people in general. So, it's difficult to put that on

> people, for me, because I don't want to make people feel uncomfortable. I don't want to make others experience a bad thing. I feel like people have enough going on in their lives and enough discomfort that they don't need to have more of that. And I also feel that, I suppose, it is my vulnerability also that makes it difficult for me to share that vulnerability with people, because it makes me feel more vulnerable, just opening myself up and talking about that. (Rory, 50s, with fibromyalgia, chronic pain, and depression)

Rory's discussion encapsulates the struggles between backstage and frontstage strategies. And while participants across the study discussed their "backstage" strategies described above, they also recognised that alleviation of loneliness needed strategies at the "frontstage"—social interactions with others (Goffman, 1959). The challenges and successes of such "frontstage" strategies are described next as participants talked about connecting with others.

Connecting with Others—The Effort of "Making the Effort"

Reaching beyond strategies internal to the mind required "making the effort" to connect with others. Jesinta, in her late teens, with autoimmune encephalitis and depression, provided advice for someone in a similar situation: "Push yourself to kind of connect with other people even if it's hard, because you're not going to regret it". The work required to do so was emphasised by many participants, using words such as "forcing" and "pushing". For instance, Ida emphasised the need to "keep pushing", viewing loneliness as an ongoing struggle to be overcome:

> Try to get as much human contact as possible. Try to go out as much as you can. Sometimes you get too embedded in your routine too. Sort of break that routine. Go out and do something or do something you haven't done, if you can do it. Yeah, just keep pushing. Never give up. Yeah, just keep pushing. (Ida, 60s, with MS)

Performative Struggles

While there was an imperative to connect, the societal rhetoric of self-reliance and independence also impeded strategies to alleviate loneliness. Many participants described how the challenge of discussing their chronic illnesses with others was weighed up against the need to alleviate loneliness. As explored in Chapter Four, the need to "put on a face" hiding signs and symptoms of illness, or "stage managing" to ensure people only see them on their best days, all impacted people's interactions with others. These frontstage strategies are described below, as is the resentment about the need to hide one's authentic, or lonely, self in order to participate socially. As Betty, in her forties, with multiple chronic physical and mental health condition says, performing in interactions and hiding her illness, is like having "a secret battle every day". This performativity is also described by Tammy and Tina:

> I get myself psyched up for dealing with it and putting on that happy face and not looking tired, making sure that my body isn't showing, trying to hide the obvious physical things that are happening. And that's just so much more effort. And then by the time I get there, it actually makes me feel resentful that, "Can't I just go out and do this?" And then I actually am resentful toward people I'm going to spend time with. So, it's just a massive deterrent. (Tammy, 40s, with MS)

> That's the problem with chronic illnesses, they're so variable. You can have good days where you feel like you can do all the things, so you do all the things, and then the very next day your body punishes you. That's when you close the door, go into your bedroom, sleep it out, and no one sees you… To please others, I would push my body. And I would look like I was doing okay, but what they wouldn't see the next day was me curled up in the foetal position, sobbing, holding a heat pack because I'm in so much agony. Because they only ever saw me on my best days when I was drugged up and all the other things to get through that day. (Tina, 30s, with multiple physical and mental chronic conditions)

Obstacles to Connection

In light of the performative struggle to perform social connection, participants talked about how they struggled to socially connect and how their chronic illness(es) impacted this. Even when they described how their health conditions contributed to their struggle, they still perceived that it was their responsibility to reduce their loneliness. Perceptions of loneliness as being socially undesirable or being a burden to others exacerbated the struggle to connect with others. For participants Laura and Rory, mental health symptoms challenged connection:

> When my anxiety is really high, I literally cannot. I can't just turn up and start talking to people or look into a room or anything like that. I can't do it. (Laura, 50s, with arthritis and bipolar disorder)

> I have a social anxiety anyway, so it's difficult for me to know when and who I can make friends with and actually putting myself out there to do it too. I do find it hard to talk to strangers, yes. I'm very much an introvert, so I really have to practise hard at just sort of putting myself out there. It's always an effort for me to do so and it's not something that comes easy to me. (Rory, 50s, with fibromyalgia, chronic pain, and anxiety)

The rhetoric that frames both loneliness and chronic illness as undesirable and burdensome to others blocked participants' initiatives to connect. Many discussed not wanting to be a "liability", or to be seen to be "whingeing", resulting in their lonely selves remaining hidden:

> It's very difficult being so down, but not being able to talk to anyone about it too much. Because I don't want to burden my friends. And also, I don't know what even to say… It's very difficult to say, "Oh, I'm depressed" (Lea, 20s, with polycystic ovary syndrome (PCOS) and anxiety)

> I don't go to my friends as much because I don't want to burden them. So I usually just go to my mum and stuff. I know at the end of the day they'll always be there and supporting me, but I just can't help but feel

> bad for them that "Oh, they have to put up with me." (Zarah, 20s, with MS and depression)

> It's very lonely when you've got pain and not well. I never used to tell the kids, because I don't think they were that interested. If they were, they would've visited me. But I never wanted them to think that I was whingeing. And there was many times I'd just cry. And sometimes one of them would say, "What are you crying for?" And I'd just say, "I don't know." I did know, but I didn't want to say that. (Cecilia, 70s, with complications after a lung transplant)

Additionally, Luke described how, even at organised events, his condition prohibited meaningful social interaction:

> I went to a few [community events], but it was very hard because I couldn't keep that communication with people because half the time I couldn't see who was there. And because there were so many people, it's hard to recognise everybody's words, which I have to rely on. I can't see facial identification at all. As I said, I only see a blob. And so, I stopped going to those as well, because I found I was just sitting there and occasionally someone might come and say hello. And I thought, "Well, I might as well stay in my apartment and be comfortable at least." (Luke, 60s, with visual impairment, chronic pain and other chronic conditions)

When Connecting Works

Some participants described the range of ways they had lessened their loneliness by connecting with others in their community. Taking on a specific role, such as volunteering, decreased the risk associated with reaching out to others. Competently fulfilling volunteer roles also "forced" participants to be sociable with others as indicated by Jessica, Adelaide and Michella:

> I immediately involved myself in the community because I didn't know anybody. So, I joined the community association. I hang out at the cafe and I chat to people. And even now, someone walks into the cafe and

> goes, "How do I get to such and such?" and I'm the one that will pipe up and tell them where to go. And on the way they might be interested in stopping in and seeing this or that, because I've done the walk or whatever. (Jessica, 60s, with MS)

> I decided that I would actually reach out to people, rather than not. And that's what's happened. I've got a good friend in the village here, I have got a little volunteer job with the local cancer support people and I go into the office and be a receptionist for three hours once a month. So I keep myself busy because I have to. If I don't, I'd be just flat. (Adelaide, 80s, with pulmonary fibrosis and osteoporosis)

> I volunteered at our local Salvo's shop. That really helped me as well, because it forced me to have to be bright and friendly to people. And I ended up really, really enjoying that. Because the same people came in each Saturday, so I was able to help them find things. And I knew that volunteering was a good strategy as well to help mental health-wise too... Because being in the shop was forcing you to be friendly and sociable, when that is something that I have found hard to do. (Michella, 50s, with systemic lupus erythematosus)

Yet opportunities to volunteer could be constrained by the uncertainties of symptoms requiring flexibility by the organisations where these volunteer opportunities were available. A number of participants expressed a desire to volunteer but were unable to due to the severity of their symptoms, while others had given up volunteering when their illness worsened.

Maintaining Positive Connections

As discussed in Chapter Four, good relationships with others are pivotal to addressing loneliness and a small number of participants talked about ensuring that they maintained their relationships with family or friends. Doing so still entailed the work of connecting described above; however, these participants described positive outcomes from their efforts:

> I realised that I'd been avoiding doing things and seeing people I love because I told myself I don't like to travel because I have PTSD and I

> get stressed and tired. So again, I was the one limiting myself and realising that helped me start to overcome it. So then I reached out to my dearest, oldest soul sister, and I went to see her and it was so beautiful, so nourishing. When you connect so deeply and intensely and beautifully with somebody who knows me so well. But not only to receive from that connection, but to give back through that connection, it was really special. (Betty, 40s, with chronic pain, musculoskeletal issues and PTSD)

> It's like me ringing my friend. I'm thinking, "I'm feeling a bit alone here tonight. I want to talk to someone," and I know that I can talk to her about silly things or we can watch TV together and talk about, you know. (Bianca, 60s, with fibromyalgia and severe food and chemical sensitivities)

> We both congratulate each other for recognising when we're not feeling well and acknowledging that and not feeling guilty and not feeling bad and kind of like boosting each other up to feel more confident in it. And I think that's actually been a huge—I've only been friends with [friend's name] for a few years, the last couple of years, and I think that's been a huge change, having somebody that can relate. (Elizabeth, 30s, chronic bowel obstruction)

Adelaide's approach to connection changed over the research process. During her second interview Adelaide described recognising that she needed to "rearrange her thinking", before making connection with others, describing how this change started when she offered a lift home to a friend:

> They would invite me in for a coffee, and then they invited me in for a meal, and we've had a couple of sessions with some board games and meals. And so, yeah, we've become quite good friends. Not in each other's pockets, but certainly from time to time. It's very nice. I'm very happy… After our last talk [interview], I found that a lot of my mental restrictions fell away and I decided that I would actually reach out to people, rather than not. And that's what's happened. (Adelaide, 80s, with pulmonary fibrosis and osteoporosis)

Adelaide illustrates here how she was able to reflect on, challenge and resist some of the expectations that had been guiding (and obstructing) her interactions with others. The freedom from expectation that she experienced from interacting with a friend, and the ability to be authentic and free from others' expectations, contributed to alleviating loneliness:

> I go and stay with my friend overnight. Yeah, we have tea together and then we'll have breakfast together and then I come back home. And I'm actually glad to come back home. I think, "Oh yes. Well, the heart's feeling okay now," because I've had that interaction. And I think, what it is, is there's no expectation from anybody about me. *They don't expect me to do anything, be anything different to what I am. And that, in itself, assuaged the loneliness that would creep up, and does occasionally, tap me on the shoulder.* (Adelaide, 80s, with pulmonary fibrosis and osteoporosis; emphasis added)

Conclusion

Our research shows that people with chronic conditions who are lonely implement strategies to alleviate loneliness and do so alongside the additional challenging context of living with chronic illnesses. While participants discussed a range of strategies, most evident in their accounts was the way dominant ideas about loneliness were reflected. They worried about being rejected, about being a burden on others and about the expectations of others. In this way, loneliness was a problem located within the individual; and participants saw alleviation of loneliness as their own responsibility, rather than as an issue of social structure, where ideas, meanings, values, along with social position shape loneliness. That participants accepted that they were responsible for loneliness, is not surprising given the high societal value placed on individualism and self-responsibility for self-care and social connectivity (Wilkinson, 2022) and the "moralist undertone" that loneliness carries (Sagan, 2023). However, the notion of self-responsibility does expose why loneliness is so challenging to address. If the actions that are taken to fix loneliness are focused on individuals only, then this is likely to create and fuel a cycle or "recursive cascade" of more self-reliance, more isolation and increasing loneliness (Manderson & Warren, 2016).

The inward facing strategies such as distraction or thinking positively were described in detail by nearly all participants and reinforce the dominant idea that change must come from within, from one's mindset. Inward facing strategies such as distraction and reframing, often conducted as "backstage" strategies, were vital to being able to undertake the work required to focus outwards to the "frontstage" of interactions. Similar to McKenna-Plumley et al. (2023) we found that connection functioned at both the internal and external levels to keep loneliness at bay, providing social support as well as being a distraction strategy. However, reaching out to connect with others was challenging for most participants. Thus, both the internal and external work—this constant effort of "making the effort" to alleviate loneliness—adds to the considerable work already associated with living with, and managing, chronic illnesses. Moreover, participants described how reaching out to other humans as being a significant act of performative work to overcome loneliness, is replete with risk. Disclosure about the experience of chronic conditions is described by participants as risking the potential gains of social interaction. With interactions being inherently performative, participants feel they must ensure that they are not a burden on others, drawing on strategies such as "masking" their true selves to successfully socially interact. It is therefore unsurprising that strategies such as volunteering changed the dynamics of social interaction, allowing participants to enact a different role, even if only for a brief time. Yet as our participants described, unpredictable mental and physical health made sustained commitment to volunteering challenging. As such, innovative or creative ways of encouraging people with illness to be able to participate, through for example flexible scheduling and diversity of activities, could encourage pathways into volunteering, even for those who experience significant chronic ill-health (Crittenden, 2018).

As we discussed in Chapter One, despite increased knowledge that loneliness is widespread, indicating that it is both part of the human condition as well as a public problem (Franklin, 2012), strategies to combat it remain largely focused on individuals rather than on community or wider social structures. However, as pointed out by Neves et al. (2023), "the 'social' is often overlooked or brushed aside as a minor dimension that the individual has the power to fully change or counteract" (p. 153). The accounts given by participants about the strategies they draw on to ameliorate their loneliness are themselves embedded within the social—within ideas about responsibility, dependence, and individualism. Their strategies are diverse and contextualised to how they simultaneously experience loneliness and their chronic conditions; however, individual agency as an antidote to loneliness is limited. As we see throughout this book if strategies to alleviate loneliness are to be effective, there must be greater acknowledgement of the relational context within which loneliness occurs including the broad range of social factors that fuel loneliness.

References

Beames, S., Andkjaer, S., & Radmann, A. (2021). Alone with Goffman: Impression management and the TV series. *Frontiers in Communication, 6*, Article 676555. https://doi.org/10.3389/fcomm.2021.676555

Bury, M. (1991). The sociology of chronic illness: A review of research and prospects. *Sociology of Health & Illness, 13*(4), 451–468. https://doi.org/10.1111/j.1467-9566.1991.tb00522.x

Charmaz, K. (1994). Identity dilemmas of chronically ill men. *The Sociological Quarterly, 35*(2), 269–288. https://doi.org/10.1111/j.1533-8525.1994.tb00410.x

Cheung, M. M. Y., Lewis, S., Raja, R., Willis, K., Dubbin, L., Rogers, A., & Smith, L. (2024). Disruption and improvisation: Experiences of loneliness for people with chronic illness. *Qualitative Health Research*. https://doi.org/10.1177/10497323241265329

Franklin, A. (2012). A lonely society? Loneliness and liquid modernity in Australia. *Australian Journal of Social Issues, 47*(1), 11–28. https://doi.org/10.1002/j.1839-4655.2012.tb00232.x

Goffman, E. (1959). *The Presentation of Self in Everyday Life*. Anchor Books

Han, M. S. W. (2022). More-than-human kinship against proximal loneliness: Practising emergent multispecies care with a dog in a pandemic and beyond. *Feminist Theory, 23*(1), 109–124.

Kharicha, K., Manthorpe, J., Iliffe, S., Chew-Graham, C. A., Cattan, M., Goodman, C., & Walters, K. (2021). Managing loneliness: A qualitative study of older people's views. *Aging & Mental Health, 25*(7), 1206–1213. https://doi.org/10.1080/13607863.2020.1729337

Kretzler, B., König, H. H., & Hajek, A. (2022). Pet ownership, loneliness, and social isolation: A systematic review. *Social Psychiatry and Psychiatric Epidemiology, 57*(10), 1935–1957.

Manderson, L., & Warren, N. (2016). "Just one thing after another": Recursive cascades and chronic conditions. *Medical Anthropology Quarterly, 30*(4), 479–497.

McKenna-Plumley, P. E., Turner, R. N., Yang, K., & Groarke, J. M. (2023). Experiences of loneliness across the lifespan: A systematic review and thematic synthesis of qualitative studies. *International Journal of Qualitative Studies on Health and Well-Being, 18*(1), 2223868. https://doi.org/10.1080/17482631.2023.2223868

Neves, B. B., Sanders, A., & Kokanovic, R. (2019). "It's the worst bloody feeling in the world": Experiences of loneliness and social isolation among older people living in care homes. *Journal of Aging Studies., 49*, 74–84.

Neves, B. B., Waycott, J., & Maddox, A. (2023). When technologies are not enough: The challenges of digital interventions to address loneliness in later life. *Sociological Research Online., 28*(1), 150–170.

Sagan, O. (2023). Organised loneliness and its discontents. *Diversity & Inclusion Research, 1*(1), Article e12008. https://doi.org/10.1002/dvr2.12008

Sagan, O., & Jones, D. W. (2024). The loneliness pandemic? *Journal of Psychosocial Studies, 17*(1), 2–14. https://doi.org/10.1332/14786737Y2024D000000014

Shi, Y., Yang, Y., Wang, L., & Zhang, J. (2023). The lived experiences of loneliness of adults with chronic conditions aging at home: A qualitative systematic review and meta-aggregation. *Geriatric Nursing, 51*, 274–285. https://doi.org/10.1016/j.gerinurse.2023.03.025

Verity, L., Schellekens, T., Adam, T., Sillis, F., Majorano, M., Wigelsworth, M., & Maes, M. (2021). Tell me about loneliness: Interviews with young people about what loneliness is and how to cope with it. *International Journal of Environmental Research and Public Health, 18*(22), 11904. https://doi.org/10.3390/ijerph182211904

Wilkinson, E. (2022). Loneliness is a feminist issue. *Feminist Theory, 23*(1), 23–38. https://doi.org/10.1177/14647001211062739

6

Bridging Connection? Digital Spaces and Communities

Introduction

Successive waves of technological innovation—the telephone, Internet, mobile devices, social media, and artificial intelligence—have dramatically reshaped how people create networks, communicate and relate to each other. Video-conferencing platforms have made face-to-face communication possible over large distances, and social media platforms have created greater awareness and visibility of the lives of others through videos, livestreams, stories and posts. Recent innovations in virtual and augmented reality are further blurring boundaries between embodied and digital connecting. Networks of 3D virtual worlds, like VRChat and Meta Horizon, are attempting to create immersive social spaces where people can interact and form communities through customisable avatars. AI-powered tools from chatbots to AI companions raise new questions about the nature and utility of digitally mediated social support (De Freitas et al., 2024; Jacobs et al., 2023; Wygnańska, 2023).

From the late 1990s onwards, digital spaces have been critical sites for support, connection and identity work for many individuals with chronic illness, as evidenced by their early adoption of these platforms (Conrad et al., 2016; Hardey, 2002). Michael Hardey's (2002) article "The

S. Lewis et al., *Unravelling the Layers of Chronic Illness and Loneliness*,
https://doi.org/10.1007/978-981-96-7909-6_6

story of my illness", examined early use of websites where people with chronic illnesses could "rewrite their biography and transform their social network" (p. 32). Digital spaces can enable the cultivation of online communities where people provide support (Kingod et al., 2017), find information and share knowledge (Maslen & Lupton, 2020; Nettleton et al., 2005; Ziebland & Wyke, 2012), develop forms of experiential expertise (Henwood et al., 2003), construct meaning around their conditions, share stories about illness experiences (Gonzalez-Polledo & Tarr, 2014) and build shared illness identities (Allen et al., 2016; Conrad et al., 2016; Elton, 2022; Marent & Henwood, 2023; Petersen et al., 2019; Rowlands et al., 2023; Schermuly et al., 2021; Wilson & Stock, 2021). Research has illustrated how digital technologies can complement or enhance traditional forms of clinical care delivery (Gherardi, 2010; Henwood & Marent, 2019; Pols, 2012), while creating new forms of solidarity through online peer support networks (Tucker & Lavis, 2019). Online spaces have also been found to be helpful for individuals to handle disclosure of illness, self-presentation and the boundaries between their illness identity and other aspects of self, with positive effects on social connectedness (Lawless et al., 2022; Petersen et al., 2020).

Yet in addition to the potential social connectivity benefits of digital spaces, there are distinct challenges and complexities associated with navigating digital spaces and technologies while living with chronic illness. Digital spaces such as social media, are spaces in which individuals with illness must balance tensions between authenticity, performativity, intimacy and meaningful connection. Navigating online relationships and self-presentation across multiple digital spaces is new identity work for people with chronic illnesses (Marent & Henwood, 2023). More broadly, as noted in Chapter Five, the immediacy and availability of social media may contribute to cultural expectations about availability and response times, creating a constant state of potential connection or "connected presence" that can be both comforting and demanding (Burchell, 2024). The work of connecting in the digital age has given rise to concerns about "digital overwhelm", "hyper-connectivity" (Candiotto, 2022) and the quality of technologically mediated relationships (Brubaker, 2022).

As we discussed in Chapter One, loneliness interventions that utilise digital technologies and platforms are increasingly popular (especially since COVID-19) and embedded in healthcare organisation and care delivery (Lupton, 2016; Petersen, 2019). Social scientists have critiqued how these technologies have often been uncritically seen as tools for individuals and healthcare providers to accomplish chronic condition self-management goals and increase healthcare delivery efficiencies (Henwood & Marent, 2019). Less attention, however, has been paid to how people with chronic illness engage with and value these kinds of technologies in their daily lives, whether they increase or erode trust in one's network, and how helpful (or not) they are in ameliorating their loneliness (Petersen et al., 2020).

Below we present participants' perspectives on the role of digital technologies, communities and spaces in the experience of loneliness for those with chronic illness, including the extent to which digital spaces and tools are seen as helping or hindering meaningful social connection. When asked about their engagement with online spaces, social media and other forms of digital connecting, only some participants reported that they engaged with digital spaces as forms of connection with others. As described below, many participants were ambivalent about digital connection or struggled to engage fully.

Bridging Distance and Staying Connected with Illness

Used as strategies to alleviate loneliness, digital platforms such as social media, online chronic illness groups, health forums, and mobile-based applications (apps) designed for social networking and connection, offered new avenues for social connection for those with chronic illness because these platforms transcend physical limitations, geographic boundaries and temporal constraints (Maslen & Lupton, 2020; Rowlands et al., 2023; Wright et al., 2023). Symptoms of illness, such as fatigue, immobility, pain and social anxiety constrained participants' access to physical spaces and their ability to stay socially engaged, rendering many confined to home for extended periods of time. As

Nick explains, the costs (physical, emotional, and financial) involved in venturing out for in-person interactions outweighed the social benefit gained from this activity. For Nick, connecting via instant messaging and social media with friends and family bridged the physical distance that illness had created and became a primary source of connection to the social world:

> … the physical getting up, getting out, and the spending of money, and the going out to a bar or a restaurant or even just a coffee, outweighs the [social] contact. So, I can lie in bed here or lie on the sofa with a cup of coffee and be chatting away and texting away and that's fine. It's easier. I'm off my feet and I'm pillowed up around the shingles pain, like I am now (Nick, 50s, with HIV, depression and anxiety disorder)

In a similar vein, Bruno emphasised that digital technologies afforded flexibility in how, when and with whom he connected; enabling him to temper how he socialised when he experienced flare-ups of symptoms, and adjust to the demands and limits of his body:

> Due to my illness, I spend a very significant portion of my time at my desk in front of a computer, and this is where I get most of my daily stimulation. When I have the energy, I very much enjoy consuming blogs and news articles to keep up to date with the broader world, as well as social media and a group chatroom (text or voice) with some of my close friends. One could consider the latter as a sort of "virtual" space in which people may casually drop in and out. (Bruno, 30s, with chronic fatigue syndrome and anxiety)

As Bruno's quote illustrates, in circumstances where chronic illness had rendered participants physically isolated, digital spaces were an important means through which they took back control of their lives and maintained connections with people in their social networks. They emphasised how digitalisation enabled them control and flexibility in how they connected, synchronously and asynchronously; these interactions could be temporally managed in ways that in-person, physical encounters could not be. Similarly, Natalia commented that online spaces were more accepting of "sporadic-ness", thus online participation could be curated to the needs of the person including the unpredictability of illness:

> It's mostly like a message board where you can just put something out there or respond to something that someone's put out there. And it's not trying to have a video call or voice call or something like that, where you're trying to have that backward and forwards conversation. It's a bit more if I've got five minutes here or it doesn't matter if the next person doesn't reply for four hours sort of thing. That sporadic-ness is a bit more acceptable ...And sometimes your contribution can just be a heart or a thumbs up or something and you're still, I guess, communicating. You're communicating with someone, "Oh, I liked that," or, "I enjoyed that," kind of thing, without it taking so much energy, I guess. (Natalia, 30s, with multiple physical health conditions)

For those for whom illness had constrained their personal agency over vast portions of their lives, being able to choose from a suite of options: "liking" or commenting on someone's Facebook post or Instagram story, listening to a podcast, connecting or lurking on message boards, in chat rooms, instant messaging, or sharing memes; helped them find ways to ameliorate loneliness that could be adjusted to unpredictable symptoms:

> I've gotten really close to some families during this [COVID-19] lock-down through Instagram and stuff, where we would just send each other jokes or videos or talk to each other over the phone and texts and stuff. So there's definitely that. Even though I haven't been able to see certain people, I feel more connected than ever. (Zarah, 20s, with multiple sclerosis (MS) and depression)

> I like sharing things that I'm interested in, whether people like them or not. And then when people put nice things on Facebook that are inspirational, I just like responding and saying, "Back at you," "Ditto," or whatever. So there is that connection there. (Holly, 60s, with urinary incontinence, chronic pain and anxiety)

Others like Betty valued digital spaces for enabling her to choose to "be as deep or shallow as I want". This was important in the context of her illness, because it allowed her to adjust the regularity and intensity of connections to her energy levels. Brief encounters when energy was low could still have a positive effect on social connectedness:

> I still have even some reluctance about phone calls, because of the things we've talked about, fear that people won't be there for me and the energy required to engage, which is why online connections are so easy. They can be as deep or shallow as I want to make them and I can spend as little or much time as I want when it's online. When it's a phone call, it's a bit more commitment. And when it's face-to-face it's more commitment, again. (Betty, 40s, with chronic pain, musculoskeletal issues and post-traumatic stress disorder (PTSD))

As Betty's quote illustrates, digital spaces could be comforting as they reduced fear of being socially rejected while simultaneously feeling that they required less "commitment". In Betty's second interview, she shared photographs of her home office and mobile phone (Images 6.1 and 6.2), which she described as: "my connection with my purpose in life".

She explained that the virtual world allowed her to "practice connection" and also allowed her the freedom to: "disconnect from other things" like work, and bring her life into more balance:

> When I have a big deadline [at work], I can get single-minded and the balance shifts away from my social life and my self-care to my work. So those areas suffer and then that one [work] gets most of my energy. (Betty, 40s, with chronic pain, musculoskeletal issues and PTSD)

In the absence of in-person sources of connection, social media had become an important source of staying connected to friends for participants, even years after they had stopped interacting with them in physical settings. For Natalia, seeing the lives of others unfold via social media, gave her "things to think about", which fostered a sense of sharing in those experiences, even when illness restricted her ability to experience them in reality. In this way, social media platforms tethered participants (albeit delicately) to a social network, and enhanced their emotional and social well-being:

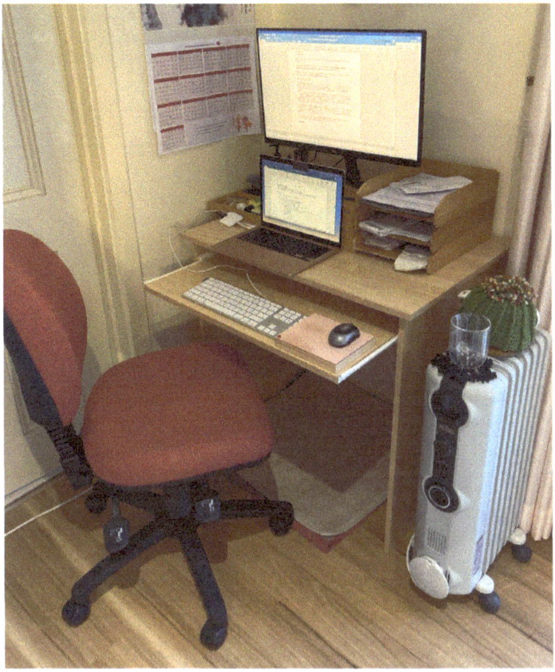

Image 6.1 Betty's photograph of her home office which keeps her connected to work and colleagues

> Even though I don't physically have people popping in for a cup of tea every day or whatever, I've got friends on Facebook that I talk to, I've got friends at work that I talk to, I've still got friends from old jobs, friends from high school, friends from this and that and the other. And I might not speak to them for six months or do more than like their photo on Facebook or Instagram or something like that, but I still feel I'm having that interaction and getting to know them and their families and that kind of thing that way. It gets you to, "Oh, that's nice." It gives you things to think about. It felt like even though, like physically, I just feel so awful - Because I'm seeing nice photos of my friends' babies or their pets or their kid at soccer or something like that, it gives you that bit of, I guess, serotonin. It gives you a smile. (Natalia, 30s, with multiple physical health conditions)

The embeddedness of digital forms of communication in everyday life was also important in reducing the sense of difference that participants

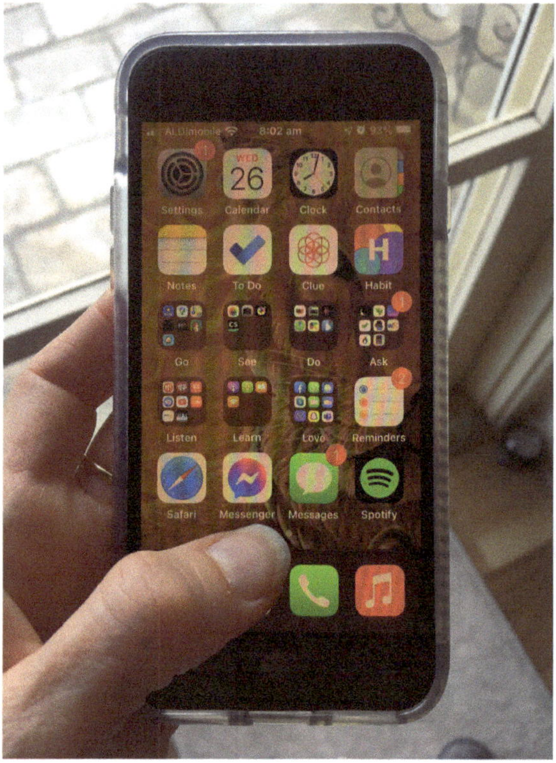

Image 6.2 Betty's photograph of her mobile phone which she uses to connect with friends through social media and text messaging

felt due to illness. Bruno, for example, described how activities that might at one time have been viewed as lonely or solitary pursuits, were now integral to social interactions for all people; illustrating how the digitalisation of social life was reconfiguring how loneliness is constructed and experienced and what activities and practices are deemed to be lonely:

> Sitting at a computer could be perceived as a very lonely activity, but with more of people's social lives migrating online, it is not so bad. (Bruno, 30s, with chronic fatigue syndrome and anxiety)

Natalia, below, similarly described how the disruption that illness had created in her life was lessened because of how embedded digital technologies had become in everyday life. The ubiquity of digital forms of social connectivity, both decreased the reliance that she and others had on seeing people "physically", but also reduced the sense of difference she felt (which, as shown in Chapter Two, is central to the experience of loneliness):

> I guess having those things [social media] be more common has made it less of a negative change, if that makes sense, because you're not relying on having to physically see people. Which works for them as well, because some of them have got social anxiety or other conditions. (Natalia, 30s, with multiple physical health conditions)

Finding New Communities Within and Outside Illness Identities

Much of the literature focuses on the social benefits of digital illness communities providing opportunities to exchange knowledge, share experiences, and provide mutual support in a safe environment (see e.g. Hardey, 2002). In our research, only a small number of participants described actively participating in online communities. Most participants, however, did value online spaces as a way to *feel* a sense of solidarity and belonging through seeing or listening to authentic stories of illness (e.g. through podcasts or social media posts), giving them "a stronger feeling of connection to the world". For Zarah, even though she did not share her own experiences of multiple sclerosis online, seeing the content that others with MS shared on social media, including their struggles and "bad" days, helped her feel less alone in her experience, and showed her that a "great life" was possible with MS.

> It's nice to relate to people. Because I think there's a trend now, where people are just showing things how it is instead of making it seem like their lives are perfect. So, some people I follow who have MS, they'll post about how they had a bad day or something, and it just makes you feel

> like you're not alone... social media helps with the MS, because I follow people who've got MS and it's nice to see how they live such great lives with such a horrible diagnosis… (Zarah, 20s, with MS and depression)

Zarah also found comfort following a church friend's social media page as she shared her experience of living with a different autoimmune condition. Her quote illustrates how people can forge peer bonds online with those who share similar experiences of chronic illness, even though they do not share the same diagnosis:

> When you see people just be raw and honest, it kind of goes, "See, I'm not." I don't know, it sounds bad, but if you're going through a tough time and someone else is going through a tough time, I don't know why, it just makes you feel like the world's not against you and it's not personal… like this comforting feeling…We're able to create this connection of we're here for each other. (Zarah, 20s, with MS and depression)

Similarly, Natalia talked about the feeling of connection she gained from listening to other people's stories of illness: "it almost feels like I'm having a conversation"; her account highlights that cultivating connectedness does not necessarily require dialogue or mutual exchange of support:

> I sort of dipped the toe into listening to podcasts. And now I listen to them all the time and I actually find there's quite a few that are about chronic illness. And even though I'm not talking to them, like the ones that I mostly listen to tend to be two people, they're having a conversation with each other, and you're listening to it, and so it almost feels like I'm having a conversation. It feels like I'm interacting with them without me actually having to. I've only got to listen, and I might think my own thoughts about what they said. But I think that's been really helpful as well, just to feel like you're listening to other people talking. (Natalia, 30s, with multiple physical health conditions)

As with offline spaces (discussed in Chapters Four and Seven), authenticity was an important ingredient in creating meaningful online connections. For the small number of participants who did engage in online chronic illness communities and groups, they told us that these were some of the only spaces where they felt that they could be open and honest about the reality of their experience. For Betty authentic relating involved sharing "what's hard" and was the basis for meaningful connectedness via social media. She describes the chronic illness online group as an authentic space, as a way to distinguish it from other "shallow" online connections, in which (as she describes below) people curate their lives in positive, aspirational ways:

> We express things quite honestly about where we're at and what we're learning about ourselves... these Facebook connections are quite honest. They're not those shallow Facebook connections where people present what they wish they were, or only talk about what's wonderful in their lives. We share what's hard and we share what we've learned. So, they're meaningful connections. (Betty, 40s, with chronic pain, musculoskeletal issues and PTSD)

Like Betty, Laura (below) was also seeking peer connections with people who shared her diagnoses online, though unlike Betty she was still in the process of trying to find a community or a space where she felt she belonged. As her quote illustrates, living with multiple complex physical and mental chronic health conditions made it much more difficult to find others with shared experiences of illness, both on- and offline:

> I'm looking for support or I'm looking like, where do I fit in?... I'm on different groups on Facebook and that, I'm on bipolar groups, I'm on personality disorder groups. Because you're trying to work out, where do you fit in? Who are my peers? Who can I talk to about this? And I don't feel at the moment, I've found anyone to talk to about it… that's where I'm finding it difficult. Yeah, because you do want to try and find people that maybe, yeah, have sort of travelled that path… We all try and find where we fit in. And you don't always know where do I fit in? (Laura, 50s, with arthritis and bipolar disorder)

Whether or not online interactions are displacing in-person connections is a matter of some debate (Brubaker, 2022). It may be the case that digital spaces enabled people with chronic illnesses to build and maintain social connections in more flexible and personalised ways, that complemented their interactions within offline spaces (Wilson & Stock, 2021). This was described by Luke, who found participating in an online group for those with visual impairments, beneficial in alleviating loneliness. Since participating in an online support group, Luke now felt more able to "push" himself to attend an in-person social gathering; something that he had not felt able to do since losing his vision. This demonstrates both how communities that start online can move into offline spaces, as well as the potential for online spaces to be non-threatening entry points into cultivating offline communities:

> Friday nights on the internet I get on with a group of other blind people. There's about, I don't know, 10 of us, and that's really good. I really enjoy that. And most of them have got guide dogs and we're going to try and catch up. And I will go. I will push myself to go, no matter how I'm physically feeling, because we're going to have a barbeque in a garden. The thing that concerns me a bit, most of them are 42 years and younger. It's a generational thing. Already, when we're on the internet, a few times they said things I had no idea what they were talking about, because different generations. But I will have a go at it. I guess it's like grasping. I do want to, because I've always been able to socially mix quite well with everyone, but I just can't seem to put in the effort anymore. I use a lot of adaptive technology. The instructor that instructs me on it, to learn, told me about it, and I thought, "Well, I've got nothing to lose," so I got onto the group. (Luke, 60s, with visual impairment, chronic pain and other chronic conditions)

Participants also found value in forging online spaces for belonging outside of their illness identities, based on shared interests or roles, such as art, music, games, or parenting. Eloise had found community through an online painting class, creating meaningful connection with others around their shared passion for art. As she describes, forging digital communities and collective identities beyond illness were particularly important to living well with chronic illness as it allowed you to "feel like you're part of something bigger" without needing to leave the home:

> That is the best and it's safe and it's here with the dog. It's great. It's [online art class] the only thing that I get excited about. And yeah, there's a focus person each week, where they live, what they're doing, if they travel. It's interesting, met a couple of war vets that are struggling with post-traumatic stress and will tell their story. And their work is incredible, absolutely amazing. Like you would never have thought of their struggle and then they showcase some of their work. So, it's just a lovely way to meet people… It's the best form of socialising that I can do. Have a chat, we've got a Facebook group, if you've got any questions. And it's what keeps me going. (Eloise, 60s, with rare neurological autoimmune condition and other chronic conditions)

Participants described moving easily between different digital spaces, presenting different aspects of themselves within each. Natalia, for instance, commented that being able to "jump" between and dip in and out of different groups (including those oriented on chronic illness), curate and present herself in different ways (for example, through disclosing or masking aspects of illness) allowed her to exercise a degree of personal agency that was not afforded to her in offline settings:

> I'm in a lot of groups, easier to jump in and out of different groups. And I've got different groups for the different things. So I've got science-based groups that I'm in, I've got cross-stitch groups that I'm in, I've got cat groups that I'm in, I've got chronic illness groups. So I've got different things that if I feel like I want to look at something I can... You can sort of do whatever you like. Yeah, what you feel like. (Natalia, 30s, with multiple physical health conditions)

As Natalia's quote illustrates, the digital world gave participants more control and agility around how they negotiated boundaries between illness identities and other aspects of self, including how they curated and presented themselves differently across a range of digital spaces.

Virtually Connecting: Helpful or Harmful in Reducing Loneliness?

Many participants—including both those who did and did not engage with digital technologies—described struggles with technology. Some expressed that they felt left behind by the pace of technology, as more community groups and activities that they had once participated in "moved online" and as digital forms of communication had become habitualised and entrenched in daily life:

> I struggle with online stuff, so I don't really join things online. I have my own emails, Facebook and YouTube and things I'll use myself, but I don't really belong to any groups… not being able to see people face-to-face really affected me. I'm not very good on Zoom. And I actually started opting out of all those things. I don't mind a telephone call, but I do not want to see myself on the camera. (Laura, 50s, with arthritis and bipolar disorder)

> I'd like to just know more to be able to keep up with it [technology]. And I've registered with the library for us both to go tomorrow and Friday maybe for half an hour, an hour, I think it is, just to brush up a bit on. Anyway, it's something, I suppose. (Lisa, 70s, with chronic back pain)

Moreover, of the participants who did discuss digital forms of social engagement, a number expressed ambivalence or mixed perspectives about the utility of digital spaces and connections in fostering social connectedness. Some like Holly, described struggles with "understanding" the rules of virtual social interaction and described instances where her attempts to forge a connection through social media had been met with social rejection or embarrassment. She described the need to "learn about the impact of texting and the impact of, what I would have thought was a way of initiating friendships"; recounting a time when she had misread a Facebook friend acceptance as a sign that the person wished for further interaction with them:

> Because of my belief or desire for connectedness, in my mind I thought, "Well, I might like to get to know them because we might be meeting

> at a christening or a family barbeque for a child's birthday," and that is a way of not just seeing a person once, but it's a way of talking. And I might send them jokes, I might send them a link. And my son then rang me and said, "Mum, stop. Don't. We know your intention is not to cause harm, but they don't like it and they don't want it." (Holly, 60s, with urinary incontinence, chronic pain and anxiety)

As Holly indicates, she lacked knowledge of the intricate social rules of engagement, or in Bourdieusian terms, the cultural capital and social experience needed to get a "feel for the game" (Bourdieu, 1990, p. 66)—to intuitively understand the rules and expectations governing interactions across various digital spaces and technologies. Others similarly described how digital spaces, particularly social media platforms could amplify as much as they could ameliorate loneliness, due to the curation of idealised versions of self—by themselves and by others. While participants were acutely aware that other people are highly selective about what they shared (e.g. their highlight reel) about themselves on social media, upward social comparisons (i.e. comparisons between themselves and someone seen to be doing better) fuelled loneliness, as this served as a daily reminder of all the things that the person could not do or the relationships that they did not have, as Tammy recounts:

> That's the sad thing about Facebook and things like those social networking things, is you think you're living a life with people, but you're not. Liking somebody's posts about their being out and doing something isn't the same as me having been there and done it myself. So, I deliberately don't even look at that. I don't want to live through other people's lives. That's not right. (Tammy, 40s, with MS)

Illustrating the complexity of online interactions and their utility in reducing loneliness, Zarah's quote (below) reveals how the extent to which social media platforms created or hindered social connection was contingent on evolving feelings and experiences of illness:

> ...at times it's definitely very positive, and then there's the times when you start to feel crappy about your own life because you see people who are overseas, living their best life, and you're at home ... It's horrible. It's a

> nightmare. But it doesn't stop me from going on. You would think that it would stop me, but it doesn't. (Zarah, 20s, with MS and depression)

As discussed in Chapter Two, cultural assumptions about worthiness and value are embedded in social knowledges about chronic conditions, and in turn, shape how participants may present themselves to others. For example, Jessica explained that while she wanted support, she chose not to join an online support group because of her fear that this was a signal to others that she was complaining about her situation or would be seen by other group members as not "badly" enough affected by illness to warrant inclusion in the group.

> I'm not interested in being on online groups because I don't want to be deemed or seen to be whinging. Because I'm really lucky, I'm still moving around. And then if I join a support group or something like that, I get nervous that I'm not as badly off as them, I don't have the right to complain or anything like that. (Jessica, 60s, with MS)

Digital spaces were governed by some of the same social expectations and assumptions about illness that regulated other aspects of social life. And yet technology was also reshaping cultural expectations about loneliness, and the social practices that were associated with social connectedness and accessing social support. Nick describes the difficulty he has in revealing to other people that he is lonely, and his preferences for instant messaging to stay connected with others. Messaging was viewed by Nick as less threatening and emotionally loaded, while reaching out for connection over the phone carried greater emotional weight—a sign that he was "in trouble" or "being dramatic":

> You need to press that button, make that call, and whatever sort of bridge you use, so whether it's the bridge of sending somebody an SMS, which is a good thing about technology, because it allows you to make the bridge without having too much of a dramatic, emotional phone call. People think when you call them with a problem, and now, because people do so little voice conversations, when you phone somebody, people think there is a problem. It might involve sending somebody a message or even

> saying something on Facebook, whatever. That sort of contact. (Nick, 50s, with HIV, depression and anxiety disorder)

The ease with which one could interact virtually was also perceived to be a double-edged sword. While creating safer and more comfortable ways of connecting with others, there were drawbacks. First, online communication had replaced in-person interactions, making it easier to avoid in-person interactions entirely. This could set in motion a self-fulfilling cycle of increasing loneliness and fear of social interaction as people became less practiced and less comfortable with engaging socially in-person, particularly for those with highly visible or stigmatised illnesses who felt the threat of the negative social gaze most acutely:

> Suddenly, you've got your TV, you've got your radio, but now you've got your internet and you've got your telephone and you've got your SMSs and all that sort of stuff. There's a new world out there. That's fine. But previously, when you didn't have that, to some extent you were almost forced to go outside to communicate with people, weren't you? If you wanted to socially interact with people, you'd have to leave. But now you can interact with people because it can be done electronically. And suddenly it's replaced everything else. I mean, you don't even have to go outside now to buy food. (Michael, 80s, with complications from a double lung transplant)

Recognising that social media was fuelling her sense of disconnection because the interactions were less meaningful and enriching, May had reduced her participation in social media:

> I deleted Instagram for a long time. Got rid of a lot of social media because I think it's worked counter-productively. I don't really think of interacting on social media being kind of meaningful interactions. (May, 20s, with rare auto-inflammatory condition)

A prominent idea across participants' accounts was that digital connection, while playing an important role in ameliorating loneliness, was not a substitute for in-person relating as they served different roles in creating belonging. As Bruno and Nick articulate:

> Meeting people in person is much more engaging than interacting online, and they are not perfectly interchangeable activities, so a mix of both is nice (Bruno, 30s, with chronic fatigue syndrome and anxiety disorder)

> Having that contact and a bit of laugh with people you know, it's good. It's being connected and disconnected at the same time... Being in contact with people online, you're not socially out of contact with people. But the physical contact and the physical interaction, it's still a desired thing. And you do miss a hug. (Nick, 50s, with HIV, depression and anxiety disorder)

Conclusion

While there was not universal engagement in online connection, digital spaces—from structured online communities which encourage active participation to passive one-sided consumption of online content—played a mediating role in some participants' experience of loneliness. These spaces enabled participants to maintain connection through illness, and form new communities both within and outside of illness identities. Digital technologies and spaces were an avenue to social connection that they could pursue from within their own homes, when their symptoms prevented in-person interactions outside the home. The asynchronous nature of connection gave participants agency over the timing and frequency of their engagement. Sharing experiences of living with chronic illness with others in similar situations provided support and validation of their experience. For some participants, their online support contributed to a sense of feeling seen, heard and understood, facilitating a sense of belonging and thus reducing overall feelings of loneliness. Similarly, other research has found that online communities can help people living with chronic illness forge deep connection and meaningful friendships with others as a result of shared understanding and empathy (Allen et al., 2016; Wilson & Stock, 2021). At the same time, online relating could also have the potential to amplify feelings of loneliness, particularly for those who compared themselves with others online who were socially better positioned, or who perceived that online relating was less meaningful or authentic than in-person, embodied interactions.

While there has been a proliferation of online interventions to tackle loneliness (Fu et al., 2022; Shah et al., 2019; Shah et al., 2021), many participants in our study expressed mixed feelings about the utility of digital spaces in accessing social support. The views expressed highlight the potential challenges of seeking to "solve" complex social problems like loneliness with technological fixes. While healthcare providers and major technology companies are increasingly investing in the development of platforms and apps to foster connection and community for people with chronic conditions, the dominance of this approach risks oversimplifying both the complexity of the lived experience of chronic illness and the multidimensionality of meaningful social connection (Neves et al., 2023). Participants' accounts suggest that in some circumstances, digital technologies may intensify, rather than alleviate, feelings of loneliness. This is especially the case for those who do not have access to the technology, energy, cognitive reserves, or the digital literacy necessary to participate meaningfully in digital communities.

References

Allen, C., Vassilev, I., Kennedy, A., & Rogers, A. (2016). Long-term condition self-management support in online communities: A meta-synthesis of qualitative papers. *Journal of Medical Internet Research, 18*(3), Article e61. https://doi.org/10.2196/jmir.5260

Bourdieu, P. (1990). *The logic of practice*. Polity Press.

Brubaker, R. (2022). *Hyperconnectivity and its discontents*. John Wiley & Sons.

Burchell, K. (2024). *Constant disconnection: The weight of everyday digital life*. Stanford University Press.

Candiotto, L. (2022). Extended loneliness. When hyperconnectivity makes us feel alone. *Ethics and Information Technology, 24*(4), 47.

Conrad, P., Bandini, J., & Vasquez, A. (2016). Illness and the Internet: From private to public experience. *Health, 20*(1), 22–32. https://doi.org/10.1177/1363459315611941

De Freitas, J., Uğuralp, A. K., Oğuz-Uğuralp, Z., & Puntoni, S. (2024). Chatbots and mental health: Insights into the safety of generative AI. *Journal of Consumer Psychology, 34*(3), 481–491. https://doi.org/10.1002/jcpy.1393

Elton, L. (2022). Knowledge, community and care: Digital biocitizenship in gestational diabetes. *Sociology of Health & Illness, 44*(9), 1408–1426.

Fu, Z., Yan, M., & Meng, C. (2022). The effectiveness of remote delivered intervention for loneliness reduction in older adults: A systematic review and meta-analysis. *Frontiers in Psychology*. https://doi.org/10.3389/fpsyg.2022.935544

Gherardi, S. (2010). Telemedicine: A practice-based approach to technology. *Human Relations, 63*(4), 501–524.

Gonzalez-Polledo, E., & Tarr, J. (2014). The thing about pain: The remaking of illness narratives in chronic pain expressions on social media. *New Media & Society, 18*(8), 1455–1472. https://doi.org/10.1177/1461444814560126

Hardey, M. (2002). 'The story of my illness': Personal accounts of illness on the Internet. *Health, 6*(1), 31–46.

Henwood, F., Wyatt, S., Hart, A., & Smith, J. (2003). 'Ignorance is bliss sometimes' constraints on the emergence of the 'informed patient' in the changing landscape of health information. *Sociology of Health & Illness, 25*(6), 589–607.

Henwood, F., & Marent, B. (2019). Understanding digital health: Productive tensions at the intersection of sociology of health and science and technology studies. *Sociology of Health & Illness, 41*, 1–15.

Jacobs, K. A. (2023). AI Companionship and Loneliness. *Humanizing Artificial Intelligence: Psychoanalysis and the Problem of Control, 51.*

Kingod, N., Cleal, B., Wahlberg, A., & Husted, G. R. (2017). Online peer-to-peer communities in the daily lives of people with chronic illness: A qualitative systematic review. *Qualitative Health Research, 27*(1), 89–99.

Lawless, M. T., Hunter, S. C., Pinero de Plaza, M. A., Archibald, M. M., & Kitson, A. L. (2022). "You are by no means alone": A netnographic study of self-care support in an online Community for Older Adults. *Qualitative Health Research, 32*(13), 1935–1951.

Lupton, D. (2016). Towards critical digital health studies: Reflections on two decades of research in health and the way forward. *Health, 20*(1), 49–61.

Marent, B., & Henwood, F. (2023). Digital health: A sociomaterial approach. *Sociology of Health & Illness, 45*(1), 37–53. https://doi.org/10.1111/1467-9566.13538

Maslen, S., & Lupton, D. (2020). Enacting chronic illness with and through digital media: A feminist new materialist approach. *Information, Communication and Society, 23*(11), 1640–1654. https://doi.org/10.1080/1369118X.2019.1602665

Nettleton, S., Burrows, R., & O'Malley, L. (2005). The mundane realities of the everyday lay use of the internet for health, and their consequences for media convergence. *Sociology of Health & Illness, 27*(7), 972–992.

Neves, B. B., Waycott, J., & Maddox, A. (2023). When technologies are not enough: The challenges of digital interventions to address loneliness in later life. *Sociological Research Online, 28*(1), 150–170.

Petersen, A. (2019). *Digital health and technological promise: A sociological inquiry*. Routledge.

Petersen, A., Schermuly, A. C., & Anderson, A. (2019). The shifting politics of patient activism: From bio-sociality to bio-digital citizenship. *Health, 23*(4), 478–494.

Petersen, A., Schermuly, A., & Anderson, A. (2020). Feeling less alone online: Patients' ambivalent engagements with digital media. *Sociology of Health & Illness, 42*(6), 1441–1455. https://doi.org/10.1111/1467-9566.13117

Pols, J. (2012). *Care at a distance: On the closeness of technology* (p. 204). Amsterdam University Press.

Rowlands, H., Aylwin-Foster, E., Hotopf, M., Rayner, L., Simpson, A., Lavelle, G., & Lawrence, V. (2023). A qualitative exploration of the psychosocial needs of people living with long-term conditions and their perspectives on online peer support. *Health Expectations, 26*(5), 2075–2088.

Schermuly, A. C., Petersen, A., & Anderson, A. (2021). I'm not an activist! Digital self-advocacy in online patient communities. *Critical Public Health, 31*(1), 204–213. https://doi.org/10.1080/09581596.2020.1841116

Shah, S. G. S., Nogueras, D., van Woerden, H., & Kiparoglou, V. (2019). Digital technology interventions to reduce loneliness in adults: A systematic review. *European Journal of Public Health, 29*(4), ckz186.294. https://doi.org/10.1093/eurpub/ckz186.294

Shah, S. G. S., Nogueras, D., van Woerden, H., & Kiparoglou, V. (2021). Evaluation of the effectiveness of digital technology interventions to reduce loneliness in older adults: Systematic reviews and meta-analysis. *Journal of Medical Internet Research, 23*(6), Article e24712. https://doi.org/10.2196/24712

Tucker, I. M., & Lavis, A. (2019). Temporalities of mental distress: Digital immediacy and the meaning of 'crisis' in online support. *Sociology of Health & Illness, 41*, 132–146.

Wilson, C., & Stock, J. (2021). 'Social media comes with good and bad sides, doesn't it?' A balancing act of the benefits and risks of social media use by young adults with long-term conditions. *Health, 25*(5), 515–534.

Wright, M., Reitegger, F., Cela, H., Papst, A., & Gasteiger-Klicpera, B. (2023). Interventions with digital tools for mental health promotion among 11–18 year olds: A systematic review and meta-analysis. *Journal of Youth and Adolescence, 52*(4), 754–779. https://doi.org/10.1007/s10964-023-01735-4

Wygnańska, J. (2023). The experience of conversation and relation with a well-being chatbot: Between proximity and remoteness. *Qualitative Sociology Review, 19*(4), 92–120. https://doi.org/10.18778/1733-8077.19.4.05

Ziebland, S., & Wyke, S. (2012). Health and illness in a connected world: How might sharing experiences on the internet affect people's health? *Milbank Quarterly, 90*(2), 219–249.

7

Feeling at Home, Having Places to Go: The Place Dimensions of Loneliness

Introduction

There is now considerable interest in how place and loneliness intersect (Bower et al., 2023), yet little is known about the importance of place for people living with chronic conditions who are lonely. Analytical attention to place can be challenging. Gieryn (2000) argues that understanding place requires attention to three features: geographic location (from the micro to macro); the material form (built or natural environment); and the meaning and value ascribed to place. Further, all three features must be considered together to understand their significance for social life. In a similar vein, place can be defined as "any environmental locus that gathers human experiences, actions, and meanings spatially and temporally" (Seamon, 2018, p. 43). Thus, while places comprise diverse physical *spaces* (consider the diversity of the built and natural environments), *places* are produced and reproduced through the meanings attached to them and the social practices that occur within them. Over time, and through patterns of repeated use and regular rhythms of routines and everyday social exchanges, one may develop an attachment

S. Lewis et al., *Unravelling the Layers of Chronic Illness and Loneliness*, https://doi.org/10.1007/978-981-96-7909-6_7

to place, resulting in an overarching identification with a specific locale (Dubbin & Yen, 2023).

Bourdieu argued that, to understand social phenomena, social events and movements, and what people do and why they do it, it is necessary to explore the social space in which they occur (Bourdieu, 2005a; Thomson, 2014). For Bourdieu, our sense of place is linked to the notion of *habitus*—our embodied individual, acquired characteristics, dispositions and styles which are the products of our social conditions. Habitus is our way of knowing the world—our taken for granted sense we have of the world, in other words, our sense of place and our sense of the place of others (Bourdieu, 2005b). However, when our social and physical conditions of existence change rapidly or dramatically (e.g. when we develop an illness that impairs our mobility or our socio-economic situation changes drastically and we have to move), our dispositions may lose coherence. In turn, our sense of place, among other things, becomes tenuous. The dynamics of place and habitus thus inform our study of loneliness and its intersection with chronic illness.

In this chapter, we examine the place dimensions of loneliness as described by participants with chronic illness, focusing on how different types of place are implicated in alleviating or exacerbating loneliness. While Oldenburg and Brissett (1982) categorised places as "first" (home), "second" (work), and "third" (places of sociability), this has since been refined and expanded. For example, third places may also comprise commercial settings and social infrastructure such as parks and other communal spaces (Jing et al., 2024; Klinenberg, 2018; Latham & Layton, 2022). As described by Heu and Brennecke (2023), these third places may also be places that "make space for loneliness", giving space for individuals to be alone if they choose and providing opportunities for engagement if they do not. Scholars such as Littman (2021) and Finlay et al. (2024) also draw attention to the perils of normative assumptions about types of place and people's capacity to freely move between different spaces. Littman proposes the notion of "collapsed places" to understand how socially marginalised groups may experience place when their movement within and between these spaces is constrained (e.g. for those experiencing homelessness or incarceration).

Participants talked about place in interviews and those who undertook photo elicitation or walking interviews were able to point out places of importance to them, or share photos of these places. Their accounts showed that home and neighbourhood can be both a source of safety and belonging, as well as a place of loneliness. Outside the home and neighbourhood, places of purpose included the workplace, as well as those institutions that are linked to the "work" of managing their chronic illnesses—such as health facilities. Participants engaged with places outside home, work and health care that can potentially "provide a sense of personal meaning and wellbeing" (Littman, 2021, p. 1229). This included casual or incidental encounters in their community, and engagement with the natural environment.

Experiences of Home and Neighbourhoods

For many participants, home was the familiar and safe place where they could manage their conditions; many used words such as refuge, safety, rest, and recharge when describing what their home meant to them. Zarah was struggling with fluctuations in her multiple sclerosis (MS) and depression, often attributing her thoughts, feelings and actions to the impact of her conditions. Zarah's participation in the research comprised interviews and keeping a diary of thoughts, feelings and events as they related to her experience of loneliness and her chronic illness. While she described in both interviews and diary how she enjoyed meaningful social engagements with friends and family, when her symptoms permitted, her diary contains recurrent notes about the need to be at home:

> Staying home was helpful and almost like a therapy for me, because it let me take things at my own pace. (Diary entry May 9th, Zarah, 20s, with MS and depression)

> I'm better off at home where I'm comfortable. (Diary entry May 10th, Zarah, 20s, with MS and depression)

In her diary she describes the significance of her room, stating in one entry that she was feeling happy because she was "relaxed and in my safe space which is my room"; and in another "my room is my happy place". In an interview she described her bedroom as being a place where she can shut out others and follow her own rules:

> I try to make it as free of as much negativity as possible and I can go there to relax. I choose who's in here, kind of thing. Obviously there's no arguments or anything, so it's just like my place, my space. Yeah, haven to me. (Zarah, 20s, with MS and depression)

Describing her home and garden as contributing to her wellbeing, Renee said:

> I can walk in here, and it's not fancy or big or anything, but I feel safe and I feel at home. (Renee, 70s, with chronic obstructive pulmonary disease (COPD))

For Nelly, the presence of a garden was integral to her housing choice:

> When I was looking to buy, everywhere I looked was units that had little gardens, which were fine, but they were all upstairs, downstairs. And at that stage my health was just starting to deteriorate and I thought, "I just want a little place with just a little garden and all on one level." And do you know, it was so hard to find. Anyway, I eventually found one. So I'm in my little house with my little garden on one level, but it was hard to find. (Nelly, 70s, with COPD)

Others, like Rosemary and Michella, shared photographs of their gardens as representations of their affinity to their homes. (see Images 7.1, 7.2, 7.3).

However, for other participants, particularly those who were socially or economically marginalised, their sense of place in the world had been disrupted. These participants described feeling dislocated from, or "out of place" in, their neighbourhoods and local communities. This disruption arose for some participants when moving to new neighbourhoods due to financial precarity. Lisa was living on government benefits and

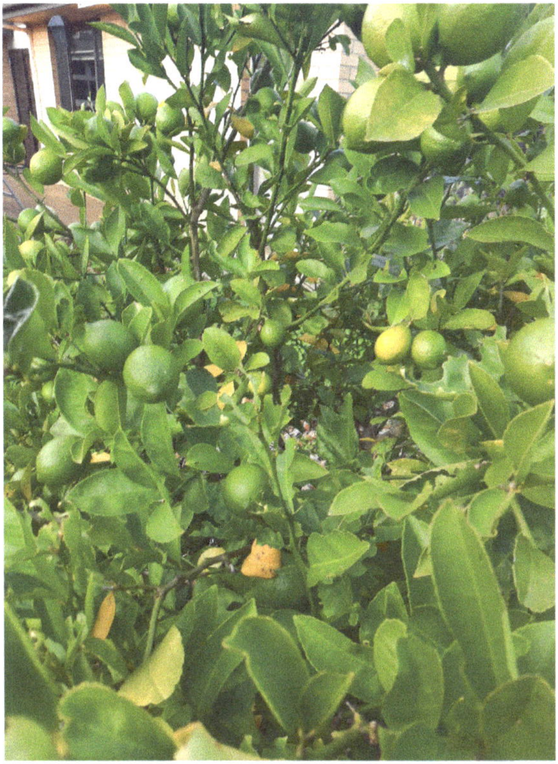

Image 7.1 Rosemary's photograph of her lemon tree

suffering from severe back pain related to injuries she sustained in a car accident. She and her husband had been priced out of their previous community and relocated to a low-income neighbourhood in a rural town. For Lisa, this strange new environment and her lack of trust in her neighbours, created feelings of fear and anxiety. She isolated herself in her home as a self-protective mechanism. For her, loneliness was the price of feeling safe:

> I don't trust people anymore. That's why I keep isolated. [I] just don't trust the neighbourhood...I have next-door neighbours; I don't know them...I like to keep to myself. I'm very aware of who comes to the door and who we speak to. We're very fussy. We've got to be, otherwise

we're not going to be safe. You feel very unsafe. (Lisa, 70s, with chronic back pain)

Jasper was living with a complex seizure disorder that meant he was unable to work. He was living in social housing with his daughter. Like Lisa, Jasper felt unsafe in his neighbourhood. In contrast to Lisa, however, Jasper had grown up in the neighbourhood where he lived. His lack of trust came from what he described as insider knowledge of the community. He described a paradoxical feeling of belonging: he "does and doesn't" belong, at once attached to place (the familiar) yet also estranged from it. His loneliness came from feeling that he is an "outsider" in the only home he has ever known. He fantasised about

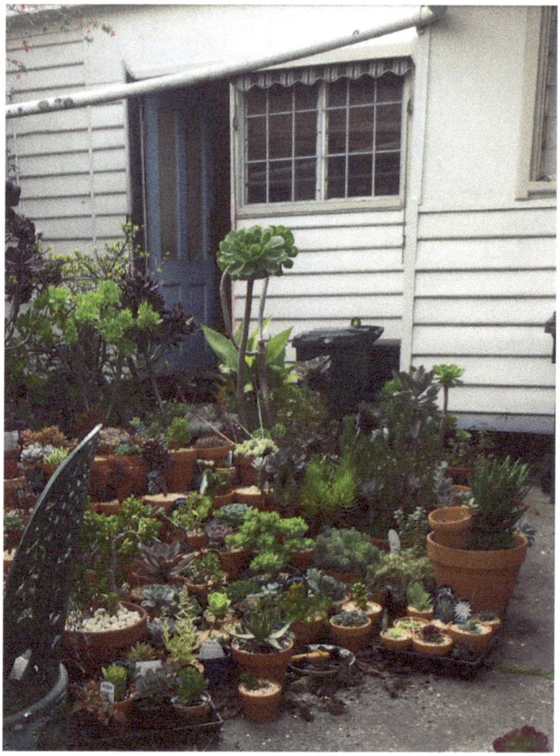

Image 7.2 Rosemary's photograph of her garden

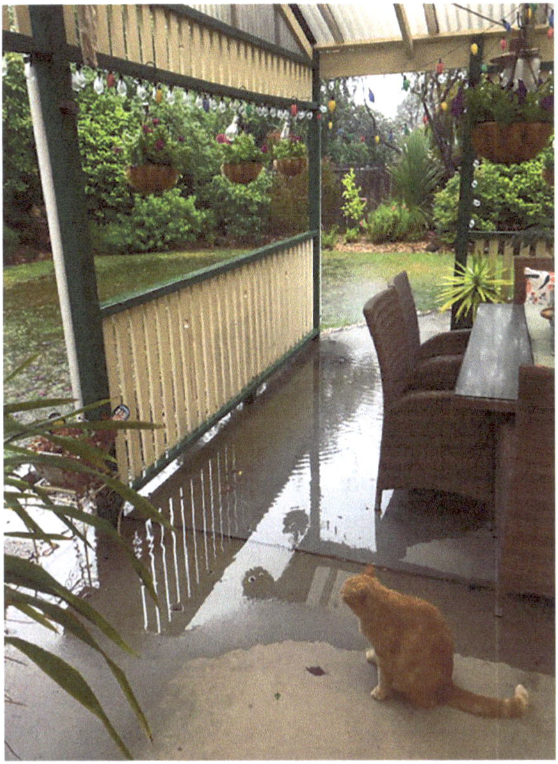

Image 7.3 Michella's photograph of her patio and garden

"escaping this place" by moving to Norway where he imagines he would belong, but his low economic capital, reliance on government housing assistance, fear of the unfamiliar and sense of duty to provide stability for his daughter, all anchor him to his neighbourhood:

> In this area, is a whole lot of public housing, all very condensed and they've got issues one way or another…they pour out of there onto the street, knocking on your door or trying to sell you drugs…half the energy is just trying to survive them. That's the synthesis of being lonely when you're in communities like this…everybody's got problems, and you can't associate with them or else you get their problems dumped on you as well. There is more loneliness here because you have to isolate. Because I

> don't want to end up on heroin or an alcoholic or falling in with riff-raff. So there's a whole lot of people, geography, demographics, and all that. It really is significant. (Jasper, 50s, with epilepsy)

Perceived crime has been identified as a cause of loneliness in disadvantaged neighbourhoods (Jamalishahni et al., 2024). For both Lisa and Jasper, their sense of dislocation in place and their drive to self-isolate was structured by their knowledge and understanding of their environment (real and imagined) and how they saw themselves in relation to others who resided there. In both scenarios, socially disconnecting from neighbours in their lived environment was self-protection that came at a cost: in Jaspers's words, this was "the synthesis of being lonely".

Fluctuating or progressing illness, combined with changes in the social infrastructure of their neighbourhood and its residents, also contributed to participants' sense of their home and neighbourhood as unstable. Verna was living alone in social housing. Her life trajectory changed dramatically when she was diagnosed with MS in her late twenties. As a young adult, she was extremely active—hiking, sailing, and travelling the world, including Antarctica. Now, she was mostly tethered to her apartment. Her loneliness was linked to the limits of her body and the physical place she inhabited. She described herself as "a woman over 55 with a chronic illness who shakes and tremors and stutters'" Beyond the physical weakness that was symptomatic of MS, her chronic illness produced a social vulnerability that contributed to her loneliness. She described how she learned to keep to herself, not trusting any of her neighbours, in such an environment:

> It was very hard here, in the beginning. It felt very dark and grim. That, this was it. I was finally dependent totally on the government. I was not able to look after myself. And then I got in here [social housing], people would knock on my door and I'd think, "Oh, that's so nice." And then I'd invite them in for a cup of tea and realise they'd nicked something…I feel I've got to keep my head down. I don't discuss anything with any of them [neighbours]. I wouldn't trust any of them as far as I could throw them. [In social housing], there's this thing of the weak preying on the weaker. (Verna, 60s, with MS)

It is in situations like Verna describes that Bourdieu's concepts of habitus and social space are evident. As Verna's experience exemplifies, while she felt at home she also occupied a challenging social space—living alone in social housing. As her physical condition declined, she found it more and more difficult to navigate her local area. Instead, she said, "I can quite happily just hunker down. Going out is difficult". Her quote illustrates how the home can be simultaneously a place of comfort and confinement.

Places for Purpose and Recognition

Having a place to go away from home was often important in ameliorating participants' loneliness and assisting them in feeling more connected—even if only temporarily. For some participants, like Michella, the structure and purpose of the workplace offered a much-needed escape from thinking about chronic illness. She revealed that going to work allowed her to maintain a professional identity outside of illness. Her attachment to the workplace was central to her life and identity as is evident in her interview and the photographs she shared of her work (Images 7.4 and 7.5):

> I don't work for money. I work for a sense of purpose, for the social contact. And I'm very good at what I do and [my boss] recognises that. And to know that somebody appreciates what you can do and somebody that can help you to grow and you could learn from [is important]. (Michella, 50s, with systemic lupus erythematosus)

These images, of how she had decorated her work pod, and the rainbows she shared with her colleague on her drive to and from work, represented the workplace (and her colleagues) as a vital source of connectivity in her life.

While Michella's connection to the workplace were related to being known outside their chronic illnesses, other participants valued places where they were known and accepted with chronic illness. Some participants who were unable to work due to their illness developed a place

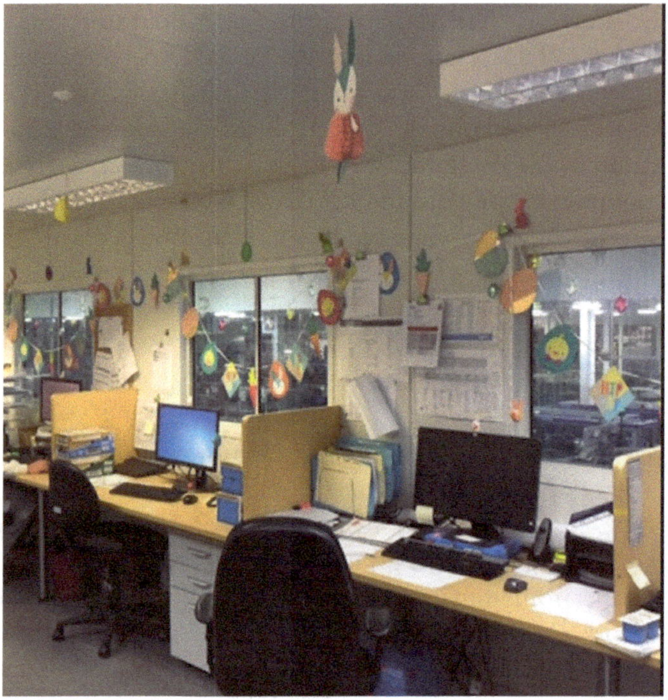

Image 7.4 Michella's photograph of decorating her workplace

attachment to their hospital, doctor's office, or community clinic. These sites featured prominently in their walking and photo elicitation interview imagery (see Images 7.6 and 7.7). Nick was living alone in a multi-story social housing tower in an inner-city area. While he knew many of his neighbours in the building, his interactions with them were limited to morning greetings and occasional check-ins when one had not been seen in a while. Nick had been living with various chronic physical and mental health conditions for many years. Of his everyday social interactions, many were centred around his illness, including regular visits to his general practitioner's (family doctor) clinic (which was close by) and to a large public hospital (a short walk away). He chose to attend the hospital weekly to collect his different medications as it afforded him a regular opportunity for social interaction with the health professionals who work there:

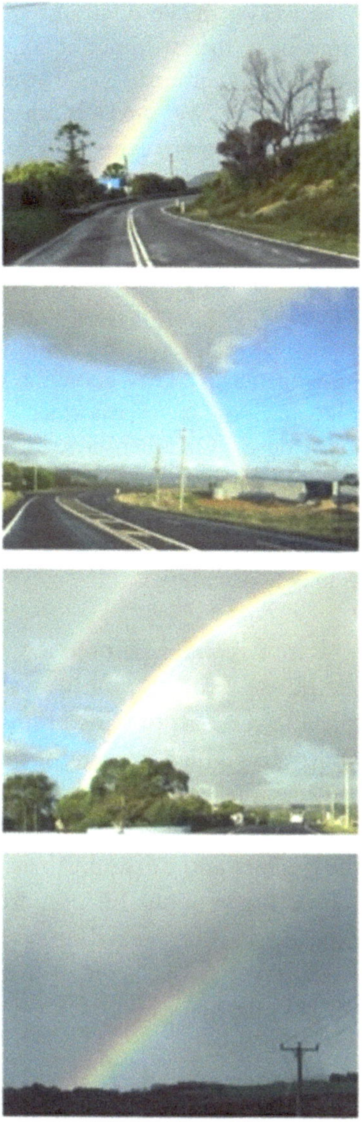

Image 7.5 Michella's photographs of rainbows during her commute to and from work

> I am very fortunate that I have [the hospital] just around the front here. I can go in and see somebody there without an appointment…There is one doctor who I've been seeing for more than 10 years and I have a very personable relationship with her. We can sit and have a chat for a really long time. They have a system over there where you can go and pick up your medications daily or weekly and I was going over once a week to top up my medications…Because of the depression and hibernating thing that I can do, I can be at home for three, four, or five days…but I was going over weekly, just so as I got out of the house, and they got to see me. I have got a good rapport and relationship with the nurses over at the clinic, and they know me. If they haven't seen me for a few weeks, so it's, "What's wrong with Nick?". They know me well enough to look at me and go "Hey, he's having a bit of a downer." Because I've walked in there and I've broken down. Or other days, I'll walk in there happy as Larry, and cheery and looking after everybody else's problems…They can sense it and they'll check. It's that checking in, "Hello, how are you?" and I'll tell them. They have certainly made a difference. (Nick, 50s, with HIV, depression and anxiety disorder)

The route Nick chose for his walking interview took in each of these sites of connection (see Image 7.6). During his walking interview, Nick explained that the clinic and the staff provided him with a sense of being cared for and cared about. His regular visits to the doctor and the hospital were important routinised social outings that gave his life structure. As his excerpt above illustrates, he highly valued the relationships that he had developed with the doctors and nurses in these spaces. He described how the staff at the clinic knew about his clinical conditions, listened to and validated his experiences, and picked up on subtle mood changes that signalled days when he's "having a bit of a downer". In knowing that they know him, Nick's feelings of loneliness were abated, even if only temporarily.

For participants who felt they needed to conceal their chronic illness in other social spheres, these medical settings gave them the freedom to be their authentic, whole selves. Elizabeth, in her early thirties, experienced debilitating bowel issues that resulted in multiple hospitalisations and frequent follow-up care. While Elizabeth still managed to work full-time, the relationship she had with the hospital staff and her medical providers

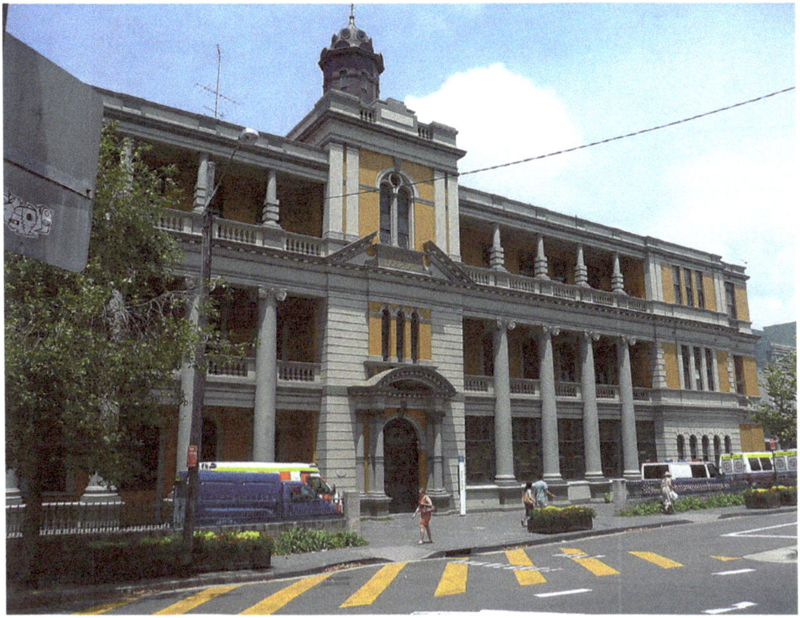

Image 7.6 Photograph taken during Nick's walking interview of the hospital where he receives monthly treatment

was a powerful mitigator of some of her loneliness. The hospital (visited during her walking interview, see Image 7.7) provided Elizabeth with a place where she need not hide her physical disabilities and where she could have meaningful and purposeful interactions with the hospital and medical staff. She described the relief of feeling safe when in hospital:

> It feels safe to me. I know it sounds silly, but it feels really safe. I know that there are people here that can help me if anything happens. I find this really comforting…and while the hospital is not some place I like to go, at the same time, it's like, if I'm going to be someplace, I'd rather be here than anywhere else. (Elizabeth, 30s, with chronic bowel obstruction)

Elizabeth was not without social support, nor did she consider herself to be alone. She worked in the healthcare field, was in a significant relationship and had a circle of close friends and family, but as shown in

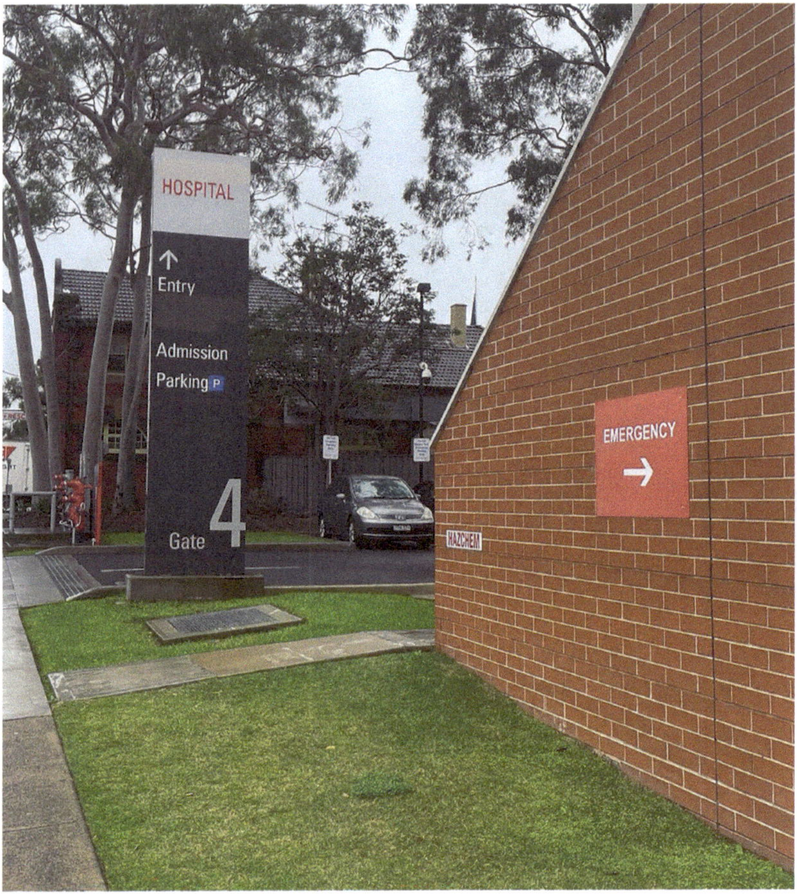

Image 7.7 Photograph taken during Elizabeth's walking interview of the hospital where she receives treatment

Chapter Four, existing relationships did not always provide the level of understanding that participants needed:

> [My friends] understand and they're very supportive, but there's not really the shared experience. My closest three friends don't really have much health stuff going on, so they don't have a huge engagement with the health system. (Elizabeth, 30s, with chronic bowel obstruction)

In contrast, with her medical team, Elizabeth could relate on a different level centring her illness and its impacts in interactions. She did not need to perform or prove anything to anyone, and her long-standing engagement with the hospital meant her expertise in her illness was recognised and incorporated into her care:

> I've had a lot of challenges still with medical doctors and around treatment and fighting about what I want and what I should be having, but knowing my own body...When I started going to [hospital] and I actually was being involved in these discussions and I was negotiating with doctors around what my treatment would look like...And now, basically I walk in and they take me seriously, they believe me. They will walk in and say, "You know what you're doing. This is what we're going to do. How does this sound? This is the plan." And I kind of back and forth with them. And then we come up with a plan and then they kind of basically say, "You're the expert. You tell us what you're comfortable with. Are we doing fluids? Are we doing food? Where do you want to go?" (Elizabeth, 30s, with chronic bowel obstruction)

Elizabeth's illness was central to her lived experience of loneliness. While friends and family were aware of her chronic illness, with them she had to engage in a mental calculus about what to share, how much to share and with whom to share it. There were no such calculations when she was in the hospital or clinic. In this environment, Elizabeth was the expert and she was confident in the knowledge she had. She was able to connect with the medical staff in a totally different way than she could with her immediate social network. Her self-knowledge, and ability to clearly articulate her medical needs and history gave her control over her illness and treatment, a more level footing with her health professionals, confidence in interacting with staff, and comfort that mitigated some of the loneliness she felt in other social spaces:

> I think that's been hugely life-changing in being able to actually engage with the system. It's a first step, but it's validated my experiences... growing more confident, but also having those positive experiences of people actually believing me. And to the point of advocating on my behalf and going further, that actually empowered me a lot, I think, to be

> able to speak up and to engage and have those conversations with health professionals that I probably would have just shied away from before. (Elizabeth, 30s, with chronic bowel obstruction)

Thus, in varying ways, places where interactions are purposeful and where participants felt valued can mitigate feelings of loneliness. They may serve as places of important social connections; but importantly, they are also places where participants feel they are legitimated and authentic. Sometimes, as in the case of Michella, such authenticity derived from her work or "non-sick" identity; whereas for Nick and Elizabeth, the healthcare setting is a place of recognition that includes, and embraces, their illness identity.

Places Outside Home, Work and Care

The third place comprises public places outside of home, work, and care that can offer "an aura of the unexpected" (Oldenburg & Brissett, 1982, p. 274). For many with chronic illness, these third places also provided an arena where loneliness could be suspended. Participants imbued value to particular places that they "felt an affinity to"—a local café, a beach, the bush, a dog park. Over time they became connected to these places and, in doing so, sometimes became recognised by others as a "normal" part of the scene, despite not being "known" at all. In research on loneliness during COVID-19 lockdowns, Klinenberg and Leigh (2024) found that such "anonymous interactions" can be particularly valuable during moments of acute loneliness. When participants engaged in these public places, loneliness was abated, if only fleetingly.

Before retiring, Ida was a hospital clerical worker. While she could no longer work due to MS, she still maintained her independence, despite living alone. At least once a week, she visited the central area of her town where she could group many activities in the same day. Through her routine, she had become recognised as part of the scene which she found immensely important in alleviating feelings of loneliness. She looked forward to the incidental social interactions she had with the local shopkeepers and the connections made there:

> I go out on Tuesday and go have lunch, maybe do a bit of shopping. You go to places that you know. It's something to look forward to...the human contact, the human recognition, like they want you to come into their shop. (Ida, 60s, with MS)

Michella was living alone in a regional area. While she was working full-time and got much joy and purpose from her occupation, she acknowledged the important role that connecting with others outside of work had on her social wellbeing. She shared a photograph of her morning walk (see Image 7.8) and said:

> I walk every morning before work. That connects me with people because there are other people that tend to do the exact same thing, at the exact same time. And even, at the end of last week, an elderly gentleman had his bin tipped over by the garbage collection and he had stuff strewn all over the street and he was saying, "I pay over a thousand dollars for a service like that." So, I stopped and helped him pick up his rubbish. And he knew straight away from the way I was walking that I obviously have hip problems. So he said, "I'm 80 and I have to have mine done as well." So, yeah, that does connect me with people. (Michella, 50s, with systemic lupus erythematosus)

The photographs taken during walking interviews, and photo elicitation frequently featured a local café or coffee shop where participants could go to feel known. During her interview, Michella shared a photograph of her coffee and newspaper taken at the local café—a place she visited regularly to connect with her community (Image 7.9). Similarly, a local café was one of only two sites for connection that Elizabeth identified during her walking interview (the other being the hospital). She said: "it's really homely, that they know what coffee you want". (See Image 7.10), illustrating the importance of being known by others.

During his walking interview, Nick took us to his local church (Image 7.11). While he does not attend the church service, he described the calming effect of its architecture, the nostalgia of hearing the bells

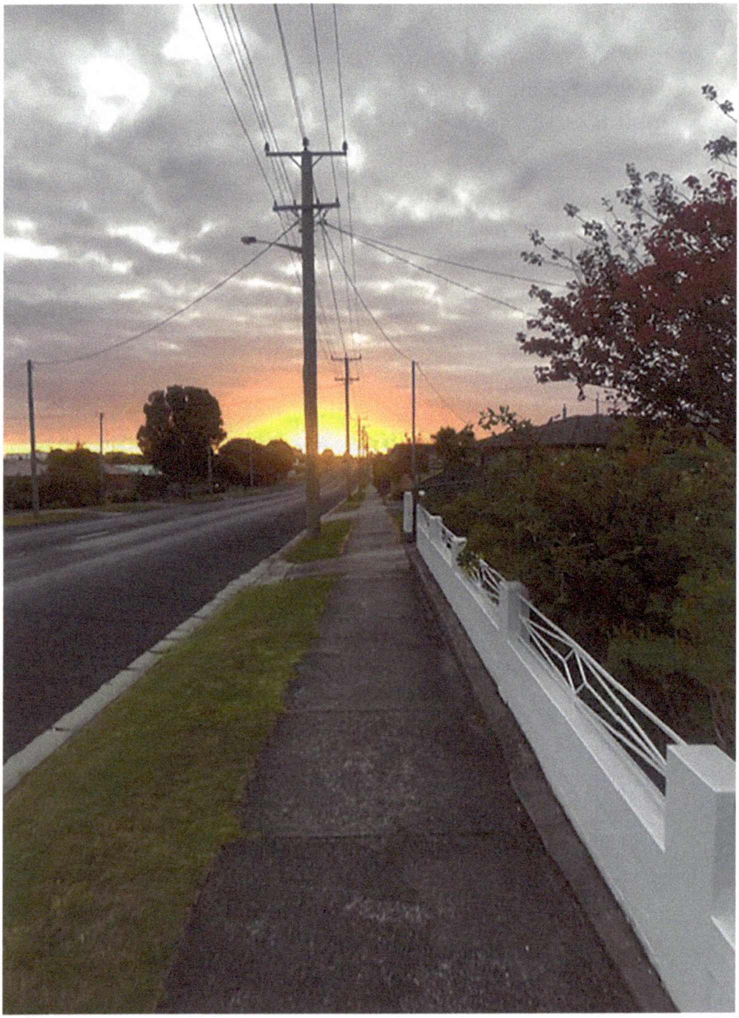

Image 7.8 Michella's photograph of her morning walk route

toll, and the comfort and safety of knowing and being known by the church caretaker. Being a short walk from his apartment, this space is somewhere he can come to feel connected:

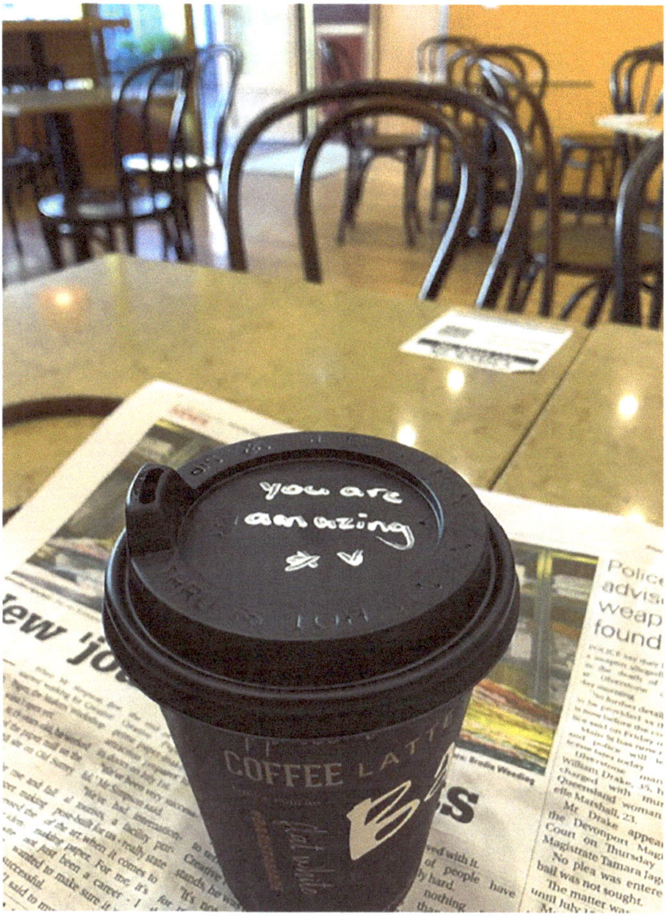

Image 7.9 Michella's photograph of her coffee and newspaper taken at her local café, a place she visits regularly to feel connected to her community

There is that safety of knowing people or knowing that there's always somebody around. The caretaker here at the church always says hello. Have I been in there? Probably about two or three times. Have I been to a church service there? Never. I'm not very churchy anymore, for lots of different reasons. But there is something for me, just walking past, there's something calming about the aesthetic of that one, about the spirituality and the history of the building. I just like walking through here. It's a nice thing… [they've] been looking after the community for a couple of hundred years. On Sundays, they still peal proper bells in here. And sometimes, I can be sitting at home on a quiet Sunday morning and I can recognise the hymns they're playing on the bells. (Nick, 50s, with HIV, depression and anxiety disorder)

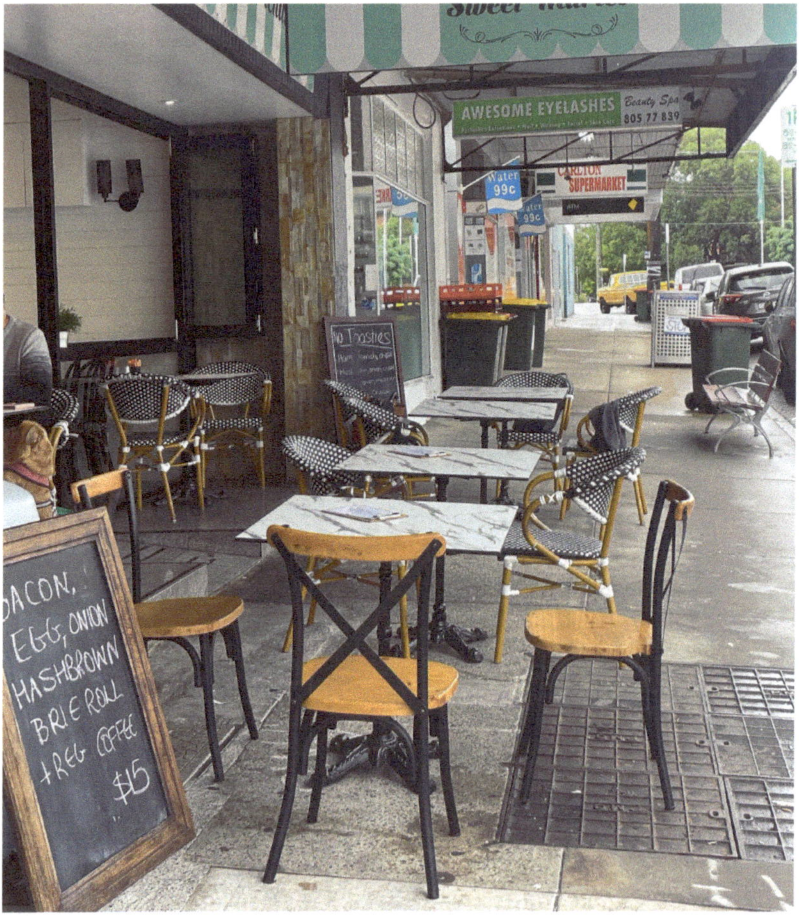

Image 7.10 Photograph taken during Elizabeth's walking interview of her favourite local café where she feels known

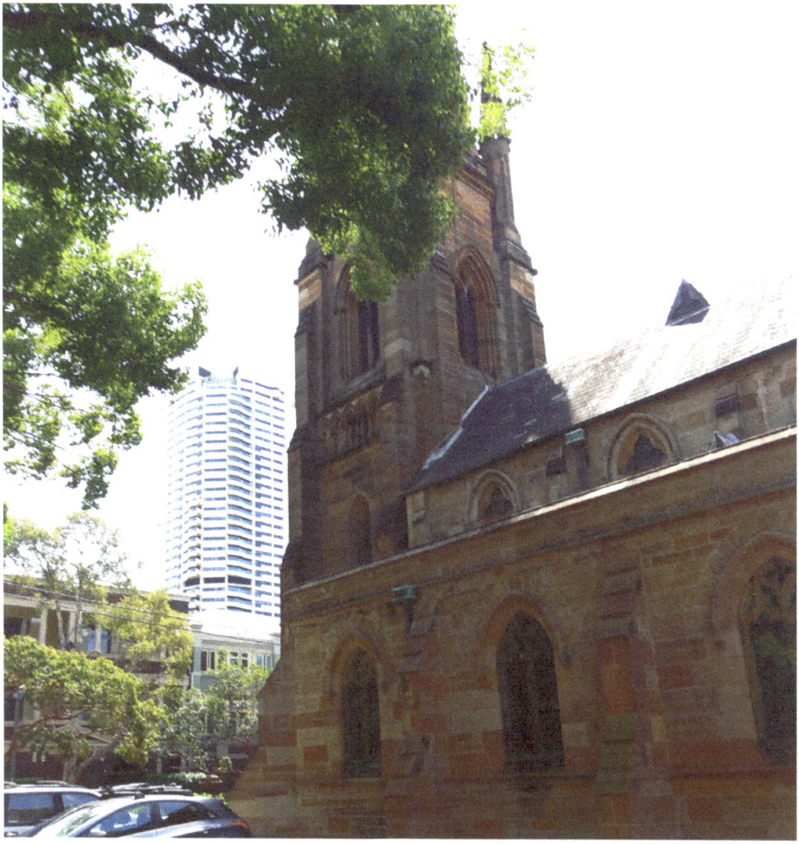

Image 7.11 Photograph taken during Nick's walking interview of the local church to which he feels an affinity

Nick, Ida, Elizabeth, and Michella all point to an important yet invisible characteristic of place that was important in ameliorating loneliness. That is, the importance of being seen and recognised as part of a community, even if one is not necessarily known. Being part of the scene contributes to a sense of belonging. It is within this dynamic and through informal contacts that feelings of loneliness, while not abated, can be mitigated. Oldenburg and Brissett (1982) assert that access to these places is not "premised on the social qualifications of the people involved" (pp. 271–272); thus, people are allowed to be different, but equal.

However, as Finlay et al. (2024) argue, the quality and access to third places is unequal. These spaces must still be navigated, and they are still imbued with broader public imaginaries of what bodies can be seen (or not seen) within them. Nicola's experiences are illustrative of the discrepancy between the ideal of the third place and the reality as experienced by someone who is "different". Nicola had found the transition to living with a chronic and, at times, debilitating illness difficult. Nicola explained that her immediate social network, while sympathetic, did not have an experiential understanding of what she was going through. On the other hand, to connect with people with MS necessarily meant exposing herself to those whose illness had progressed and were living "an unbelievably shit life". A shared understanding of illness came at a cost that Nicola found overwhelming: "[When you disclose things], you start to subtract more from your identity…you lose the choice over how people can see you and your abilities". For Nicola, the local gym had become an important space for belonging that helped her manage loneliness. She valued the ease of the incidental interactions that she had in the space and the structure it provided. She stated:

> [I] quite like having those random interactions where there's no commitment, you've got no personal investment, and that's okay, because no one really gives that much of a fuck about the other person, so there's no real consequence". [I like] the routine factor as well. I like that you have a class timetable and you start to get familiar faces. I don't necessarily know these people well, but it's just familiar faces kind of thing, and so you can have that bit of a conversation. (Nicola, 30s, with MS)

Despite feeling she belonged in this setting, Nicola had found that there were subtle ableist social rules that governed some third places like her local gym, which can make people with disabilities and illnesses, including herself, feel that they do not belong. While Nicola was "grateful" that she was "not a walking advertisement" for MS, she was reflective of her own precarious position within her third place, coloured as it was by living with a progressive chronic illness:

> I have noticed that when people can't do the activities or some of the class exercises, there isn't really a level of accommodation and it's disheartening. I've heard some people complain that sometimes when diverse people need some extra help, it distracts from the instructor's attention to the class. So when you hear mainstream people complain about shit like that, it's a bit disheartening. And these people obviously don't know that I have MS, and I don't think that they would say those things to me if they knew. It's kind of like an "us and them" mentality. (Nicola, 30s, with MS)

The natural environment (also known as green and blue spaces) was also an important third place that participants described as meaningful in ameliorating their loneliness. There is emerging evidence about the positive impacts on the physical and mental health of natural outdoor environment (Gascon et al., 2017; Smith et al., 2021), and nature-based social interventions to ameliorate loneliness are being conducted (Litt et al., 2024). For those participants who were able to access them, these places were appreciated:

> I need to walk every day in the bush. I connect with the bush. (Jessica, 60s, with MS).

> I live near a massive nature reserve, and I try and go there once a day. And it's actually quite nice to see other people out and about walking their dogs. (Nicola, 30s, with MS)

> And there's lots of farms. It's surrounded by farmland. And we have the farmlands on one side and the sea, the bay, on the other. It really is lovely. Beautiful scenery. (Adelaide, 80s, with pulmonary fibrosis and osteoporosis)

> I actually go to dog parks with support workers to have a try specifically for my mental health. So they know especially if I'm having a bad day,

> take me out to a dog park and I'll sit there and I'll watch the dogs or play with the dogs or talk to the dogs because that's what helps me. (Laura, 50s, with arthritis and bipolar disorder)

> When I go and clean [name] place, she's close to Mountains and the view is spectacular. And sometimes I just stop from the top of her place just to look at the view. It's very beautiful. (Holly, 60s, with urinary incontinence, chronic pain and anxiety)

Parks, nature reserves and other green spaces, were also important sites that people chose to take photographs of during their walking interviews, as the images taken during walking interviews with Verna (Image 7.12) and Lea (Image 7.13) and photo elicitation with Rosemary (Image 7.14), and Jessica (Image 7.15) show.

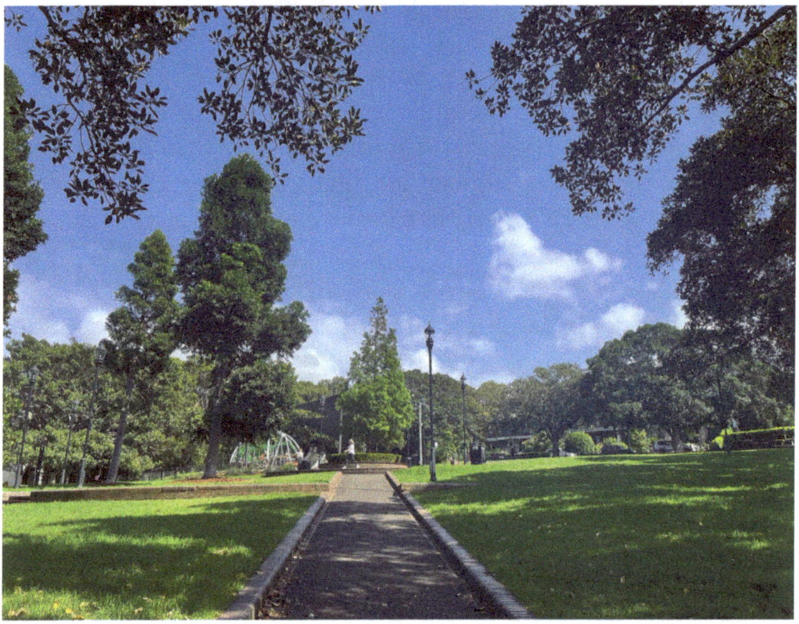

Image 7.12 Photograph taken during Verna's walking interview of her local park

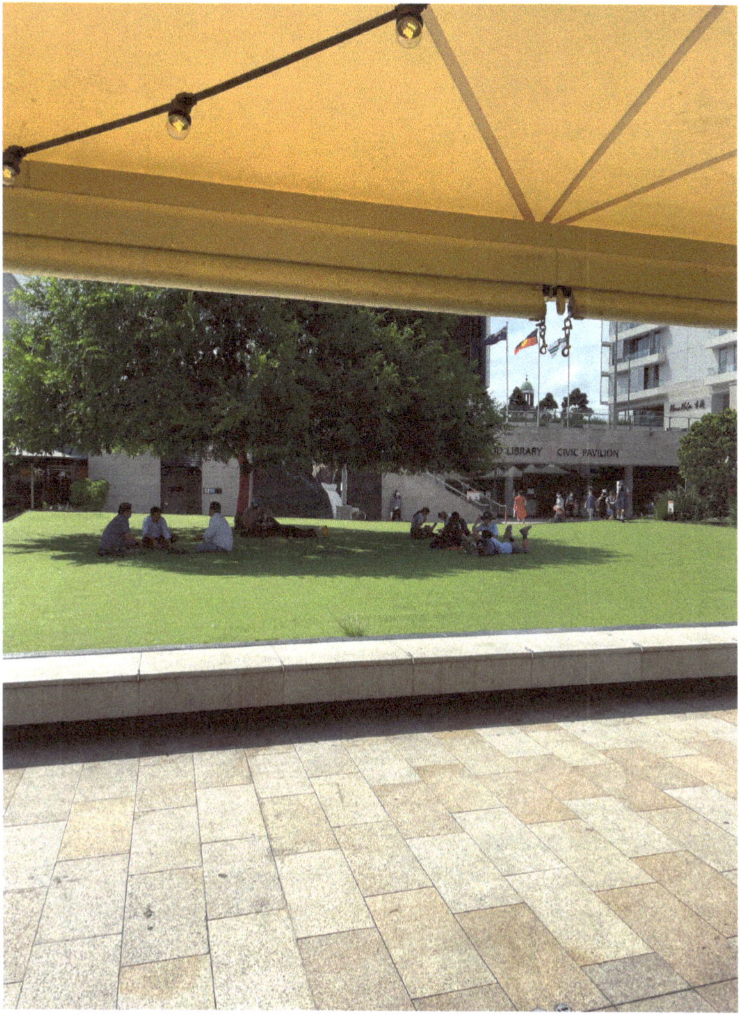

Image 7.13 Photograph taken during Lea's walking interview of a green space outside the local library where she sometimes studies

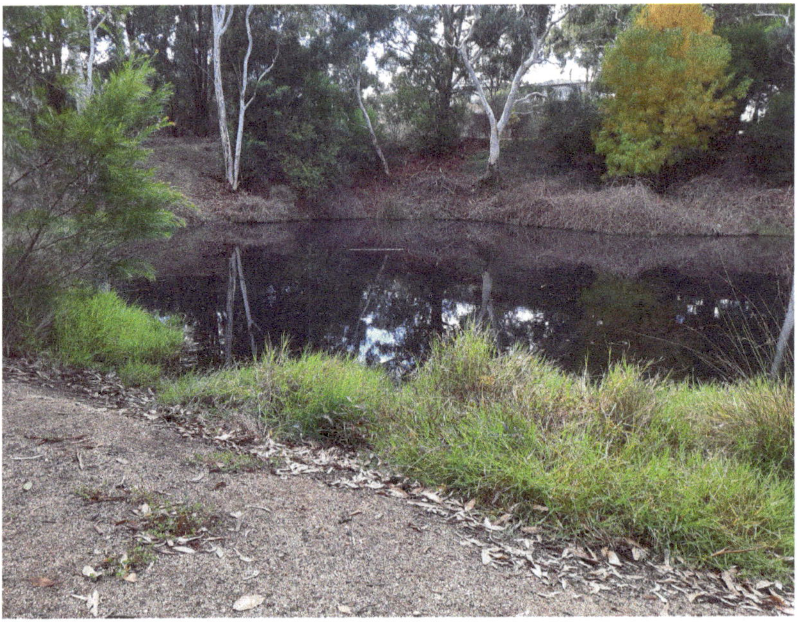

Image 7.14 Rosemary's photograph of her local dam which she describes as a place she feels connected to

There are, however, physical challenges in navigating such spaces, and for some participants their illness severely limited how they were able to access and be within these spaces. They did, however, seek to connect with these spaces in different ways. For example, Bruno, while not being able to exercise in his local park, had found driving, an alternative way of connecting with the natural world in a way that overcame the spatial and temporal constraints of his illness.

> While I am lucky enough to live close to a nice public park, I am unfortunately unable to exercise, and cannot make full use of it. I suppose the next best thing, which I also happen to enjoy, is going for a drive somewhere. I can sit by myself, take in the world outside my window as it passes by, listen to music, and since the time it takes to reach my destination is more or less fixed, I don't feel like I'm in a rush. (Bruno, 30s, with chronic fatigue syndrome and anxiety)

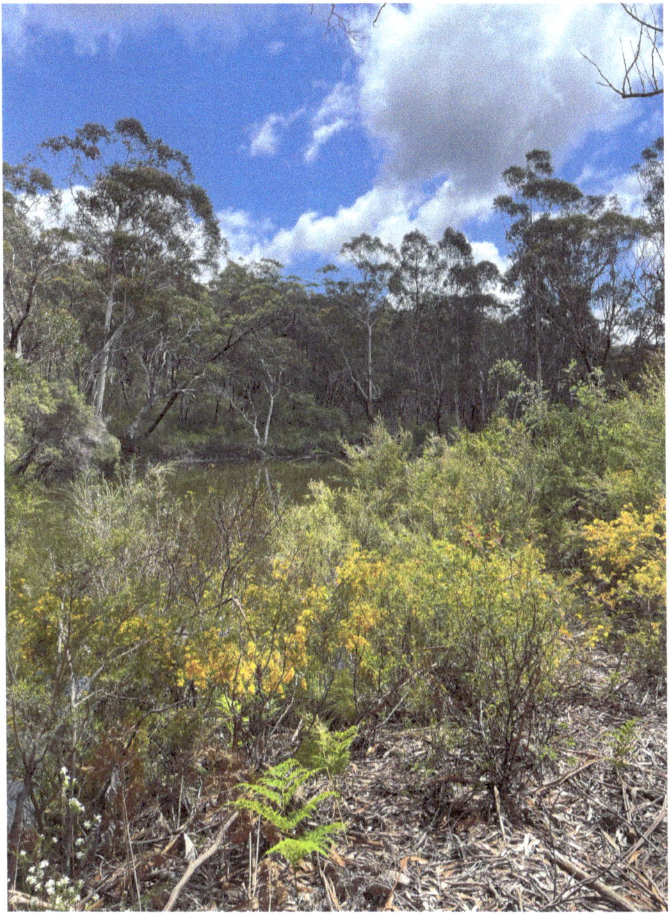

Image 7.15 Jessica's photograph of the local bushlands where she connects with nature

Greg was living with chronic pain from a back injury. At various times, he was homeless, living in his van at a local and popular beach. This beach was where he spent much of his youth surfing and he described it as his "safe place". It was the place he knew best and felt most at home.

While he recognised the beauty of the beach was integral to his sense of connection, it was the social interactions with others in this place that provided his life with vibrancy and diminished his sense of loneliness; no matter how short or superficial those interactions were:

> I am accepted at the beach. I talk to a lot of people. But the cohesive factor is the surf. We talk about the swell, the tide and the winds, and what break was here. So, there is community. But at the same time, they all go home and I never get invited, so I don't know how real that is. (Greg, 60s, with chronic back pain)

While his surfing knowledge and expertise fuelled Greg's ability to make personal connections with others that were vastly important to his sense of belonging, the boundaries of those interactions were limited to this place only. Mitigating his loneliness was therefore dependent not only on the context of this specific place, but also the transient nature of others in this space. Connections made here did not translate into other spaces, such as the home, and Greg was never invited to participate in a friendship activity outside of this beach environment.

Yet these natural places were powerful sources of connectivity, even in the absence of other people. Ross talked about his "psychological connectedness" to his local beach: "It would be hard for me to leave it... if I can't come down here and walk along the beach and sit here, I drive past the point". All of the photographs taken during his walking interview centred on the beach, as shown in Image 7.16. Others like Rosemary, also shared photographs of blue spaces that gave them a sense of comfort and belonging (Image 7.17).

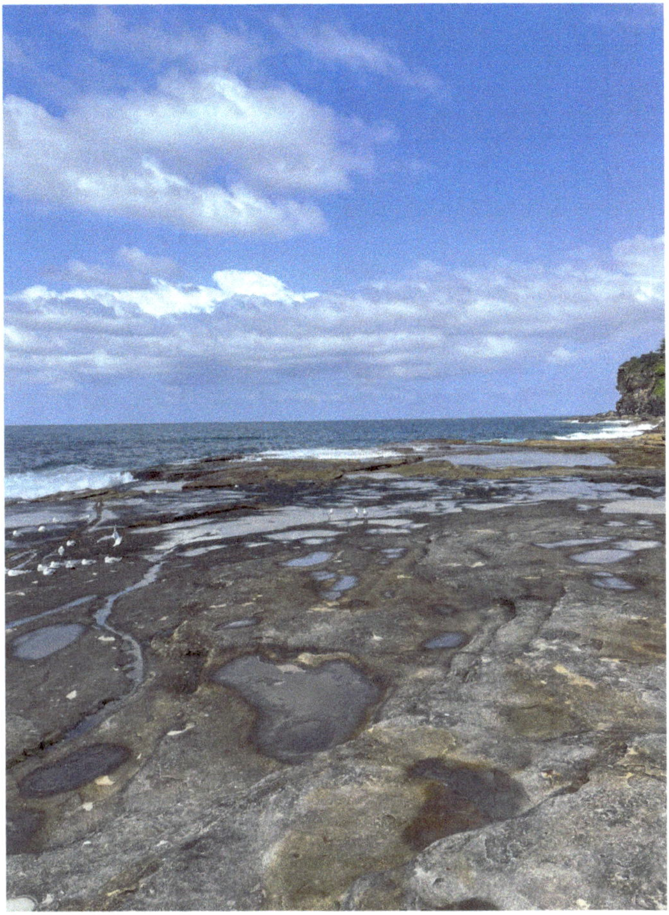

Image 7.16 Photograph taken during Ross's walking interview at his local beach, a place with which he describes a psychological connection

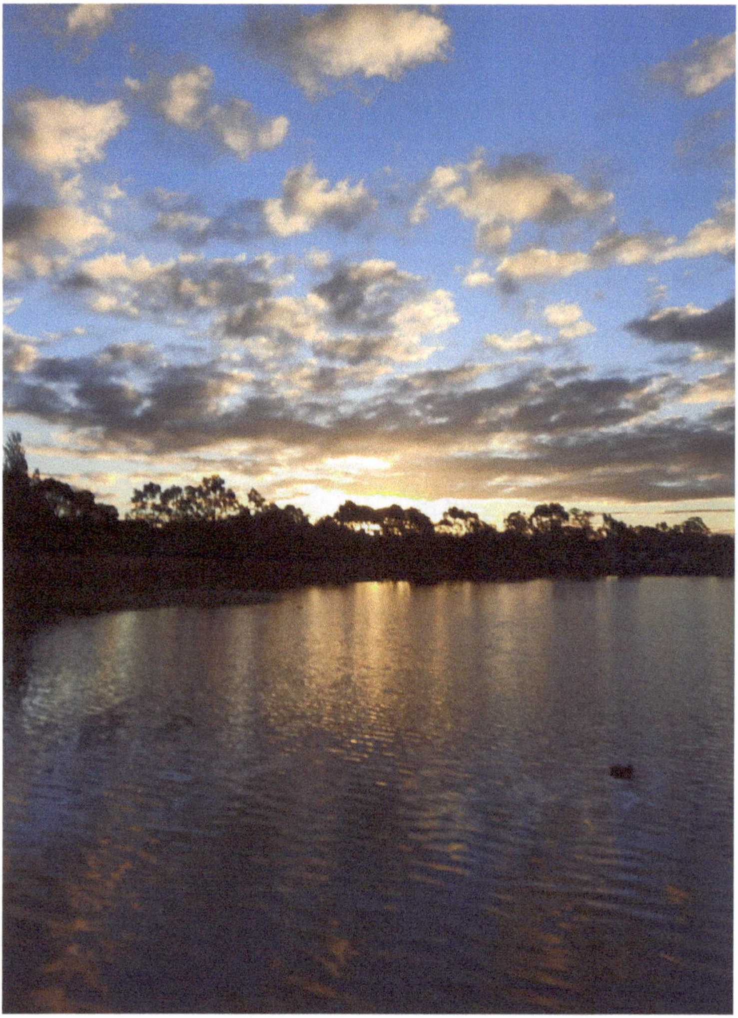

Image 7.17 Rosemary's photograph, taken at her favourite place at her favourite time of the day, representing connection to nature

Conclusion

Place and one's sense of place were embedded in the experience of loneliness for people with chronic illness. More than a combination of physical elements and characteristics, places had diverse properties and functions that either exacerbated or ameliorated the experience of loneliness. Participants' homes as refuges and places of safety could be disrupted when they feel out of step within their lived environment. Financial and housing precarity combined due to chronic conditions, and factors such as low levels of trust in neighbours, feeling unsafe and changes in housing were all disruptors that coalesced to exacerbate loneliness. The stories told by Lisa, Jasper and Verna, highlighted how economic and social vulnerability impacted and exacerbated loneliness.

Having places to go and feel seen also warded off loneliness and fostered a sense of connectedness. For participants, places for purpose extended beyond workplaces, to include health facilities. Medical places helped participants to feel less lonely because they afforded regular, predictable and safe social contact (even if it was instrumental), in ways that allowed them to exercise agency; they could choose how and when they participated in these spaces. They also provide structured social scripts with clear roles and reasons to interact, and there were social norms and expectations baked into these environments that made it easier for people with chronic illness to move within them. These medical settings were some of the only places where participants' illness identities were highly visible, and where they did not need to engage in the invisible labour of hiding the impacts of illness (as they did in other spaces like workplaces or social settings). The clinic or hospital therefore functioned as a social space where expectations differed from social or friendship settings and the authentic self, illness and all, could just be. Attachments to these healthcare settings where people felt safe, cared for and cared about, were important in fostering connection.

Likewise, engagement in third places could temporarily alleviate feelings of loneliness. Importantly, these places alleviated loneliness through being seen, being recognised or being part of the scene, even when participants were not known. It is through being in these places, where fleeting incidental interactions could occur, that there was a tacit acknowledgement that one belonged. These "ad hoc" social encounters sometimes evolved into more routinised, long-term connections that had significant social value in alleviating loneliness—albeit temporarily. At the same time, some of these places were also experienced as intimidating or discriminatory for those with chronic illness, as they struggled to navigate them physically and socially.

Throughout participant accounts, place was inextricably linked not only to the experience of loneliness but also to the compounding effects of chronic illness. Place provided meaning and solace but also displacement and disengagement. Examining the role of place in the context of loneliness and chronic illness adds another layer of understanding to the literature and healthcare practices, illuminating the complex and interwoven relationships between place, loneliness and chronic illness experiences. Place also brings to light the day-to-day efforts people living with chronic illness and loneliness have to go to in order to live well. The incorporation of place in research on chronic illness and loneliness points to the need for a broad approach to this issue and reveals the possibilities for designing innovative approaches to supporting those who are lonely and live with chronic illness.

References

Bourdieu, P. (2005a). *The social structures of the economy*. Polity Press.

Bourdieu, P. (2005b). Habitus. In J. Hillier & E. Rooksby (Eds.), *Habitus: A sense of place* (pp. 43–49). Ashgate.

Bower, M., Kent, J., Patulny, R., Green, O., McGrath, L., Teesson, L., & Rugel, E. (2023). The impact of the built environment on loneliness: A systematic review and narrative analysis. *Health & Place, 79*, 1–15.

Dubbin, L., & Yen, I. H. (2023). Renovating space to age in place: Experiences of elderly residents living through public housing renovations and reflections from affordable housing developers. *Journal of Aging and Environment*. https://doi.org/10.1080/26892618.2023.2280961

Finlay, J., Cannon, M., Meltzer, G., & Yeh, J. (2024). Aging in third places. In M. Cutchin & G. D. Rowles (Eds.), *Handbook on aging and place* (pp. 221–239). Edward Elgar Publishing Limited.

Gascon, M., Zijlema, W., Vert, C., White, M. P., & Nieuwenhuijsen, M. J. (2017). Outdoor blue spaces, human health and well-being: A systematic review of quantitative studies. *International Journal of Hygiene and Environmental Health, 220*(8), 1207–1221. https://doi.org/10.1016/j.ijheh.2017.08.004

Gieryn, T. F. (2000). A space for place in sociology. *Annual Review of Sociology, 26*, 463–496.

Heu, L., & Brennecke, T. (2023). By yourself, yet not alone: Making space for loneliness. *Urban Studies, 60*(16), 3187–3197.

Jamalishahni, T., Davern, M., Villanueva, K., Turrell, G., & Foster, S. (2024). The contribution of objective and perceived crime to neighbourhood socioeconomic inequity in loneliness. *Health and Place, 85*, Article 103165. https://doi.org/10.1016/j.healthplace.2023.103165

Jing, J., Dahlberg, L., Canter, D., & Plater-Zyberk, E. (2024). The role of third place concerning loneliness in the context of ageing in place: Three neighbourhoods in Stockholm. *Health and Social Care in the Community.* https://doi.org/10.1155/2024/4172682

Klinenberg, E. (2018). *Palaces for the people: How social infrastructure can help fight inequality, polarization, and the decline of civic life*. London: Penguin.

Klinenberg, E., & Leigh, J. K. (2024). On our own: Social distance, physical loneliness, and structural isolation in the COVID-19 pandemic. *Social Problems, 71*(4), 1216–1230. https://doi.org/10.1093/socpro/spad003

Latham, A., & Layton, J. (2022). Social infrastructure: Why it matters and how urban geographers might study it. *Urban Geography, 43*(5), 659–668.

Litt, J. S., Coll-Planas, L., Sachs, A. L., Rochau, U., Jansson, A., Dostálová, V., & Pitkälä, K. H. (2024). Nature-based social interventions for people experiencing loneliness: The rationale and overview of the RECETAS project. *Cities & Health, 8*(3), 418–431. https://doi.org/10.1080/23748834.2023.2300207

Littman, D. M. (2021). Third place theory and social work: Considering collapsed places. *Journal of Social Work, 21*(5), 1225–1242.

Oldenburg, R., & Brissett, D. (1982). The third place. *Qualitative Sociology, 5*(4), 265–284.

Seamon, D. (2018). Merleau-Ponty, Lived body, and place: Toward a phenomenology of human situatedness. In T. Hunefeldt & A. Schlitte

(Eds.), *Situatedness and place. Multidisciplinary perspectives on the spatio-temporal contingency of human life* (pp. 41–66). Springer.

Smith, N., Georgiou, M., King, A. C., Tieges, Z., Webb, S., & Chastin, S. (2021). Urban Blue spaces and human health: A systematic review and meta-analysis of quantitative studies. *Cities, 119*, Article 103509. https://doi.org/10.1016/j.cities.2021.103413

Thomson, P. (2014). Field. In M. Grenfell (Ed.), *Pierre Bourdieu: Key concepts* (pp. 65–79). Routledge.

8

Loneliness of Care, Care for the Lonely

Introduction

Loneliness not only affects those with chronic illnesses, but also those family members and other informal carers who support and provide care for a person living with chronic ill-health—referred to in this chapter as *carers* (Gray et al., 2020). Research shows that loneliness is prevalent among carers of people with chronic illnesses, such as dementia and severe mental illness (Bonin-Guillaume et al., 2022; Guan et al., 2023; Liao et al., 2024). These studies have largely focused on the loneliness experiences of older carers and/or spouses—less is known about those who provide care at different life stages or relationships. Providing care for someone with chronic illness places considerable demands on carers. Identities and roles change. Additional roles and increased responsibilities on carers can negatively impact their social interactions. They may lose touch with friends, family members, and social groups, and withdraw from social activities. Yet, while carers may experience estrangement within some relationships, the social bonds with others may become closer, demonstrating the complexities of the loneliness experience for carers (Winkler et al., 2014).

S. Lewis et al., *Unravelling the Layers of Chronic Illness and Loneliness*,
https://doi.org/10.1007/978-981-96-7909-6_8

Carers' loneliness is also tied to feeling solely responsible for the person's care and their sense of powerlessness and helplessness to change the situation (Vasileiou et al., 2017). Carers can feel restricted from social participation and more alienated from the "outside" social world. They may choose not to attend social activities without the person they are caring for as they do not want to leave them at home alone; or they may feel reluctant to accept help or respite from others. Feelings of loneliness are associated with a sense of one's own social life being "put on hold" to prioritise the needs of the person with chronic illness (Chistell et al., 2023; Davies et al., 2019).

Experiences of loneliness (for the carer and care recipient) are embedded in their social relations (Chatoo & Ahmad, 2008). Carers can experience loneliness in their relationship with the person with chronic illness due to loss of companionship, shared interests and lack of meaningful interactions (Fee et al., 2023; Greenwood et al., 2019). This may be due both to changes in the personality of the individual with the illness, or to changes in the dynamics and roles of the two people, such as increased dependency of one person on the other (Chistell et al., 2023).

Part of carers' work is negotiating boundaries between dependence and independence (Chatoo & Ahmad, 2008). They may downplay or hide their care work to preserve the chronically ill person's sense of independence and reciprocity in the relationship (Breheny & Stephens, 2009; England & Dyck, 2011). Paradoxically, this can create disconnection in the relationship when the person with chronic illness cannot "give back". A close social bond between carer and care recipient, however, can partially buffer against the negative consequences of loneliness (Willis et al., 2020). Sociologists have theorised about why some carers/care recipients with illness grow closer and some more distant, suggesting that ambiguity about the condition and greater uncertainty about how long they will be caring for is associated with a more disconnected relationship (Olson, 2016).

Societal expectations of carers, such as being stoic, accommodating, devoted and supportive, can lead them to engage in "emotion work", whereby the presentation of an outward display is not in step with one's inner feelings (surface acting) or the person tries to change their inner feelings to comply with social expectations (deep acting) (Hochschild,

1983). The need to perform a role that feels inauthentic can evoke loneliness. And when these efforts fail, carers can feel socially alienated (Wharton, 2009). The need to maintain a social interaction that feels inauthentic places the social bond under strain. There are also societal shifts in the configurations and character of family life, as well as changes across health and social care systems that mean family members are expected to take on more of the work of caring for those with chronic illness, including the work of socially supporting them. These macro-level shifts are fundamentally changing experiences of loneliness and its consequences.

In this chapter, we focus on the experiences of the family members and other informal carers who provide care and support for people with chronic illness who are experiencing loneliness. Drawing on interviews with 27 people who were caring for a person with chronic illness and experiencing loneliness (see Table 2 in Appendix), we detail how loneliness is experienced within the relationship, how relations between the carer and the person with chronic illness impact on the experience of loneliness for both parties, and with what consequences.

Filling a Social Need

Carers in our study identified that supporting a person with chronic illness who is also lonely comes with complex expectations. In addition to supporting the person to navigate their chronic illness, carers talked about the extra responsibility they felt to support the lonely person to feel more socially connected. They described needing to fulfill multiple social roles in the lonely person's life, in the absence of other meaningful social relationships. All said that they devoted considerable time to nurturing their personal connection with the person, as Cindy described:

> He really enjoys it when I listen to his music, and we sit down and sing the lyrics or dance. So, I connect with him in that way. And I book trips away and music concerts that he enjoys so there's something to look forward to and that we can share together. (Cindy, 50s, caring for son with epilepsy and autism)

However, carers found it challenging to navigate these different identities and roles simultaneously (e.g. being carer, parent and friend), because each role was governed by different expectations, as is illustrated by Jason:

> It's very difficult to draw the line between carer, therapist, father, husband, friend. I'm still the same person, but I'm acting in different roles, doing different things at different times. And trying to separate that out, it's very difficult, near on impossible. (Jason, 40s, caring for children with anxiety disorder and autism)

As the below quotes from Cindy and Vivian illustrate, knowing that they were the sole interpersonal relationship in the person's life weighed heavily on them:

> What happens if I get sick or I die and he thinks I'm the only person? That's a huge responsibility. (Cindy, 50s, caring for son with epilepsy and autism)

> Without me she would be alone and that there wouldn't be anybody to support her. (Vivian, 50s, caring for mother with diabetes and other chronic health conditions)

At the same time, carers recognised the importance of supporting the lonely person to establish their own social connections and networks. They described directing considerable time and effort to this enterprise, acting as a social conduit or "cheerleader" for the person by seeking out social groups or activities for the person, attending or engaging in these social activities with them, or including them in their own social outings:

> I try and include her in things that she might like here. There was a pride festival about a weekend ago. I took her along to that. Not ideal to go along with your dad. If she gets invited to things, I make sure I can get transport or I can drop her off. We're always on the lookout for little things to do. (Henry, 60s, caring for daughter with anxiety disorder and autism)

However, carers also reported that the person's chronic illness and its physical, emotional and social impacts, such as pain, fatigue, social anxiety, and stigma, impacted their efforts to socially support the person, as is illustrated by Rosalind:

> I try to make suggestions. I can drive him here or there or does he want to go for a drive or down to [beachside suburb] for fish and chips, for example, or whatever. But he doesn't really like going out in public. He's never really been a going out and eating type of person anyway. But he doesn't like going out that much now because he's very self-conscious of being in a wheelchair. (Rosalind, 60s, caring for ex-partner with spinal cord injury, and multiple chronic health conditions)

Similarly, Yvette disclosed that her life was tightly interwoven with that of her adult daughter. She attributed this to the physical and emotional limits of her daughter's illness that constrained her capacity for social interaction and participation. Her daughter was heavily reliant on Yvette for social connectedness and support but, as shown below, what to the outside observer appeared to be a freely chosen and close friendship, was imposed on mother and daughter by both the demands of the illness and the stigma associated with it:

> People do think that my daughter and I just hang out together. Because obviously a lot of what we do is and has to be social and sociable and whatnot, like the walking every day or going to the movies, whatever, social outings. A lot of people just think, oh, we're just doing things together. And that's because I deliberately make it look like that, because my daughter doesn't like to be seen as being sick or having a disability. (Yvette, 60s, caring for daughter with chronic fatigue syndrome and movement disorder)

Missing Out

Feeling primarily responsible for meeting the social needs of the person experiencing loneliness meant that many participants neglected their own needs for social connectedness. Many participants described themselves as profoundly lonely, as illustrated by Juliet:

> I felt very lonely. I turned to quite a few different support lines, sometimes late at night, because I just wasn't doing well, having to stay home, ... it actually really affected my mental health. (Juliet, 20s, caring for partner with fibromyalgia and polycystic ovarian syndrome (PCOS))

Carers attributed their loneliness to losing valued identities (outside of being a carer), losing valued interpersonal relationships (beyond the relationship with the person they were caring for), missing out on meaningful social activities due to their all-encompassing and all-consuming carer role, and not feeling understood by others. Cindy, introduced above, described how her interpersonal relationships had been strained because her friends did not understand her situation, the complexity and unpredictability of her son's condition, and the need to prioritise her son's welfare over her own desire for social connection:

> I've lost a lot of the people along the way who don't understand or don't want to know... every day is very different. A good day is that we can keep our appointments and we can get out of the house, and a bad day is everything gets cancelled and I just stay at home with him, next to him, whatever he requires to get through that day. There's many times where I would love to have company, but I can't invite people over here or I can't leave the house because of where [son] is at. (Cindy, 50s, caring for son with epilepsy and autism)

A unifying thread across carers' accounts was that in their caring role, they were deprived of the type of social interactions that they desired, articulated here by Larissa:

> I do have too much social interaction, but it's not the social interaction that I want... I have heaps of social interaction because I schedule our

appointments, I go to the pharmacy and do all the shopping. But my favourite thing is to be alone in my house and I'm never alone in my house ever. My gold standard of social interaction is going down to the art gallery. If I'm going into the paid exhibition, I'll talk to the person that I'm buying my ticket from, I'll talk to the person that I'm buying a coffee from. I might talk to other people in the exhibition. So... all of that kind of just incidental social interaction. That's my favourite social interaction. It doesn't sound like it's meaningful, but it's what I crave. (Larissa, 50s, caring for partner with chronic migraine)

Yet participants felt powerless to change their situation. The guilt of excluding the lonely person, or leaving them alone, obstructed participants from socialising with others, as illustrated below by Henry and Victoria. As they discussed, time and energy spent on other social relationships or social pursuits took time and energy away from the person they cared for:

> … the buck stop stops with you. There's no one else is gonna pick up. There's no one else going to be able to help…You have to put what you wanted to do aside… you can't leave the person by themselves. (Henry, 60s, caring for daughter with anxiety disorder and autism)

> There's not a lot of free time, and then when there is a bit of time, if you spend it away, then you feel guilty for being away from that person who's then stuck at home, so then you don't tend to spend a lot of time away. It is hard to balance the wife and carer role. And one's obviously a choice and the other is like a requirement almost. (Victoria, 30s, caring for husband with lymphoma and post-transplant complications)

Loneliness in the relationship was also tied to reciprocity. Larissa described how the shift from partner to carer had fundamentally changed the relationship from one of mutuality to one of increasing one-sidedness:

> You can't have one person for everything, that's not healthy. Now that I'm his carer and it's so dominating, I don't have people anymore. So he still takes a lot. I'm super independent, and he is a clinger. That worked before he got sick. That was okay. It still took more work on my part

> than his, but there could be balance. Whereas now there isn't. A number of my friends have fallen by the wayside. (Larissa, 50s, caring for partner with chronic migraine)

As Larissa describes above, taking on more of the practical and emotional work of caring for her partner meant that not only the relationship between her and her partner suffered, but her relationship with friends and others in her social network also suffered. The pressure to meet all the lonely person's social needs created an undercurrent of tension, shame, frustration, and occasionally resentment for some participants, like Rachel and Ella:

> There's a part of me that has resented aspects of it, because it was not in my life plan. (Rachel, 50s, caring for adult son with schizophrenia)

> I know being a carer shaped who I am today, but it just always felt like I never had the freedom just to explore and be reckless and carefree... there can be shame or guilt attached to thinking about yourself. (Ella, 20s, caring for brother with auditory neuropathy and attention deficit hyperactivity disorder (ADHD))

Closeness in the relationship and what one participant referred to as "hyper-dependency" rendered both parties more disconnected (from each other and their wider social networks). A recurrent theme across carers' narratives was that they felt lonely in the relationship with the person they cared for. They attributed their loneliness to feeling disconnected from their own life and other relationships, as well as feeling trapped, because of the increasing unevenness of the relationship with the chronically ill person:

> ...there's definitely loneliness that comes with not seeing other people in those social interactions, but then there's also that loneliness of it's not the relationship that you thought you would have. So it's loneliness in two different ways. (Victoria, 30s, caring for husband with lymphoma and post-transplant complications)

> I wish I could just run away. I'm ready to go move somewhere unannounced and just start a new life, where no one knows who I am. Just reset. (Ella, 20s, caring for brother with auditory neuropathy and ADHD)

Over time, participants said that they found themselves increasingly socially alienated and lonely in their experience of being a carer. For example, Victoria described how, as the person she cared for became increasingly dependent on her for social support, it became more and more difficult to separate herself from the person she was caring for and carve out her own distinct identity and social life.

> You just sort of feel isolated, like you're the only person that understands what's going on and you're in a situation that nobody else is in. Although, that's not true of course. There are other people doing the same thing and feeling the same way. (Victoria, 30s, caring for husband with lymphoma and post-transplant complications)

Vivian went on to share that the work of socially supporting the lonely person felt especially burdensome because it was unseen and unappreciated by others, particularly by the person who they were caring for:

> I found it challenging that she won't acknowledge my help. People say to her how lucky she is to have me to help her and support her. She won't acknowledge it. So sometimes I feel taken for granted. (Vivian, 50s, caring for mother with diabetes and other chronic health conditions)

Supporting the Carer

Carers described being proactive in accessing support to alleviate their own loneliness. They developed a range of strategies to help manage the experience of caring for a person with chronic illness experiencing loneliness. These strategies included practising positive self-talk, allowing themselves time for self-care activities like going to the gym, having a coffee with a friend, reaching out to trusted friends, partners, or family members, volunteering or joining a carer support group. Across these strategies, the idea of "giving oneself permission" was prominent:

> I try to validate my own feelings because it is a lot and I go through a lot. So, I allow myself to feel that way. And then I'm like, "Right, I've had my sook, I've had my cry. Put my big girl pants on. Let's go. (Audrey, 30s, caring for husband, children and mother, all with multiple conditions)

> I do train with a personal trainer...I'll leave the house. It's 1/2 an hour to [the gym], an hour with my trainer, half an hour home, maybe a little bit. And he will let me have that time now. (Larissa, 50s, caring for partner with chronic migraine)

> I've volunteered a lot in the community. I work as a carer advisor, which is only one hour a fortnight but it keeps me in the loop and connected…I started volunteering at the local church to make up food hampers for people in the community. (Cindy, 50s, caring for son with epilepsy and autism)

Yet, while carers said that these personal strategies were helpful, they also talked at length about the need for additional community or organisational supports, and initiatives to remove barriers that carers face in accessing support, such as cost and stigma:

> There's supposedly lots of resources and amazing stuff to help and support carers. Like, that's a lot of bullshit. What carers need is another 500 bucks a week. I don't need legislation to say that I should be able to have my own life, but I don't have the resources to do that. (Larissa, 50s, caring for partner with chronic migraine)

> …a lot of that requires me to reach out to them. And sometimes that's too hard. It might be helpful if there was a register or I don't know, something to say that you're caring for this person. And somebody with some sort of knowledge or whatever, on the condition initiates contact, something like that, I don't know. That might make it easier, because when you've got so much going on through your head, the last thing you do is think about yourself. (Esther, 60s, caring for child with multiple sclerosis (MS))

Ensuring that social connection is recognised and "valued as a real need" at a societal and institutional level was also seen as important. Many carers said that more work was needed to break down negative stereotyping and cultural silences surrounding "loneliness" (in much the same way as mental health) that get in the way of people disclosing that they are lonely:

> It's avoidance. If systems and services and professionals are avoiding the word "lonely", of course, how is the consumer or the carer going to bring that up? It's not valued as a real need… I think we need to break down the shame and the stigma and the myths around loneliness as well, that it's okay. Like we've said now, it's okay to talk about mental health. Well, we also need permission to talk about loneliness and to work out some really practical ways that we can really connect. (Cindy, 50s, caring for son with epilepsy and autism)

Some participants were critical of what they perceived to be an "overemphasis" on being offered support that was oriented towards helping them to be "a better carer", rather than towards their own social wellbeing. Others felt that the support that was offered to them was out of step with their needs, and oriented towards overly simplified "quick fixes" to a complex issue:

> I feel like people just flippantly go, "Oh, just join a group," or, "Just go and join some group and meet new people." I know they mean well. (Josephine, 30s, caring for partner with multiple conditions)

> Everything these days seems to be centred around social media. But social media isn't people with people… something which I feel we're all missing out on, is ways in which to help ourselves, because helping ourselves empowers ourselves as well, but we're not given any of those opportunities to help ourselves. (Jason, 40s, caring for children with anxiety disorder and autism)

Finally, the invisibility of carers (the work they do, the person they are, the loneliness they experience), pervaded all aspects of the caring experience. This sense of being unseen, undervalued, and "taken for granted"—by the person they cared for, by their wider social networks, and by the broader healthcare system—is articulated below by Alice, a long-term carer for her husband:

> Their world becomes small and it's about them. So the sicker he got, he couldn't see, and I suspect he actually didn't want to see how exhausted I was… that constantly meant even my small needs were not appreciated, acknowledged, let alone met… I felt unappreciated and taken for granted by [husband], by his family, his friends, by the health and the medical system. I felt invisible and ignored. Very few people asked me how I was. (Alice, 50s, caring for husband with MS and depression)

Alice's statement that "very few people" inquired about her illustrates how one's identity outside of being a carer can be erased or invisibilised. Similarly, Larissa observed that the thoughts and feelings of carers, including their loneliness, are forgotten or ignored because they are not recognised for their own personhood:

> It's easy to ignore [carer's loneliness] because carers are not considered individual people… You get your pension, whatever, but that role is not acknowledged. (Larissa, 50s, caring for partner with chronic migraine)

Alice went on to describe how this sense of lost identity also extended into what she envisioned for her future. Her loneliness was tied to grieving the dissipation of hopes and dreams for the future:

> At first I had hope, but over time you just lose hope. There's no hope… It's not a marathon, it's years' worth of marathons. That's what it feels like. It also feels like my losses are not seen or appreciated. I've lost a husband. I've lost my future. (Alice, 50s, caring for husband with MS and depression)

Acknowledgements and recognition in the context of caring for someone navigating chronic illness and loneliness—both predominantly invisible conditions—were critically important to help them feel more supported, as Rachel describes:

> It was the women in my life who acknowledged and believed me when I said I was dealing with what I was dealing with. (Rachel, 50s, caring for adult son with schizophrenia)

Conclusion

The perspectives of people who care and support those who are lonely and experiencing chronic ill-health provide a different, yet complementary, viewpoint on the interplay between chronic illness and loneliness. While experiences were contingent on age, gender, the duration of care, the nature of the relationship and the illness, some commonalities were evident across all carers' experiences. A universal experience was the double burden of responsibility felt by carers to: (1) support the person to manage their chronic illnesses; and (2) help ameliorate their loneliness. This sense of responsibility to fulfil multiple social roles—partner, friend, confidante, advocate, carer, connector—was both internally felt and externally reinforced by others in their social networks, healthcare professionals, the broader care sector, and within wider cultural scripts about caregiving. The moral duty to be the primary (often sole) figure of social support meant carers ultimately often sacrificed their own social needs, leading them to also feel lonely. Thus, these findings show how loneliness can move within and across the carer/care recipient relationship, and how loneliness can be experienced by both parties separately and in mutually dependent ways.

These carers' stories reveal critical gaps in how we support carers including the need for resources and supports that are personalised to carers and their needs, rather than being primarily oriented towards supporting them to be a "good" carer. They also support the need for interventions that move beyond a focus on the individual and work at the micro-level of the carer/care recipient interaction. Personal strategies for carers, while important, may be limited due to the unique barriers that are placed on carers that restrict them from interacting with others. Moreover, structural changes—both practical (e.g. respite services) and societal (e.g. social appreciation of carers' value and contribution), are desperately needed as part of our effort to ameliorate carer loneliness and support them in their carer roles.

References

Breheny, M., & Stephens, C. (2009). I sort of pay back in my own little way: Managing independence and social connectedness through reciprocity. *Ageing and Society, 29*(8), 1295–1313. https://doi.org/10.1017/S0144686X09990134

Bonin-Guillaume, S., Arlotto, S., Blin, A., & Gentile, S. (2022). Family caregiver's loneliness and related health factors: What can be changed? *International Journal of Environmental Research and Public Health, 19*(12), 7050. https://doi.org/10.3390/ijerph19127050

Chatoo, S., & Ahmad, W. I. U. (2008). The moral economy of selfhood and caring: Negotiating boundaries of personal care as embodied moral practice. *Sociology of Health & Illness, 30*(4), 550–564. https://doi.org/10.1111/j.1467-9566.2007.01072.x

Chistell, F., Stängle, S., & Fringer, A. (2023). Loneliness is a monotonous thing: Descriptive qualitative research on the loneliness of caring relatives. *BMC Nursing, 22*(1), 161. https://doi.org/10.1186/s12912-023-01327-4

Davies, N., Walker, N., Hopwood, J., Iliffe, S., Rait, G., & Walters, K. (2019). A "separation of worlds": The support and social networks of family carers of people with dementia at the end of life, and the possible role of the internet. *Health & Social Care in the Community, 27*(4), e223–e232. https://doi.org/10.1111/hsc.12701

England, K., & Dyck, I. (2011). Managing the body work of home care. *Sociology of Health and Illness, 33*(2), 206–219.

Fee, A., McIlfatrick, S., & Ryan, A. (2023). 'The care circle consists of me'. Loneliness and social isolation for older male spousal care-givers. A qualitative study. *Ageing & Society, 43*(3), 706–723. https://doi.org/10.1017/S0144686X21000854

Gray, T. F., Azizoddin, D. R., & Nersesian, P. V. (2020). Loneliness among cancer caregivers: A narrative review. *Palliative & Supportive Care, 18*(3), 359–367. https://doi.org/10.1017/S1478951519000804

Greenwood, N., Pound, C., Brearley, S., & Smith, R. (2019). A qualitative study of older informal carers' experiences and perceptions of their caring role. *Maturitas, 124*, 1–7. https://doi.org/10.1016/j.maturitas.2019.03.006

Guan, Z., Poon, A. W. C., & Zwi, A. (2023). Social isolation and loneliness in family caregivers of people with severe mental illness: A scoping review. *American Journal of Community Psychology, 72*(3–4), 443–463. https://doi.org/10.1002/ajcp.12698

Hochschild, A. R. (1983). *The managed heart: Commercialization of human feeling*. University of California Press.

Liao, X., Wang, Z., Zeng, Q., & Zeng, Y. (2024). Loneliness and social isolation among informal carers of individuals with dementia: A systematic review and meta-analysis. *International Journal of Geriatric Psychiatry, 39*(5), Article e6101. https://doi.org/10.1002/gps.6101

Olson, R. E. (2016). *Towards a sociology of cancer caregiving: Time to feel*. Routledge.

Vasileiou, K., Barnett, J., Barreto, M., Vines, J., Atkinson, M., Lawson, S., & Wilson, M. (2017). Experiences of loneliness associated with being an informal caregiver: A qualitative investigation. *Frontiers in Psychology, 8*, 585. https://doi.org/10.3389/fpsyg.2017.00585

Wharton, A. S. (2009). The sociology of emotional labor. *Annual Review of Sociology, 35*(1), 147–165. https://doi.org/10.1146/annurev-soc-070308-115944

Willis, P., Vickery, A., & Symonds, J. (2020). "You have got to get off your backside; otherwise, you'll never get out": Older male carers' experiences of loneliness and social isolation. *International Journal of Care and Caring, 4*(3), 311–330. https://doi.org/10.1332/239788220X15912928956778

Winkler, M., Bedford, V., Northcott, S., & Hilari, K. (2014). Aphasia blog talk: How does stroke and aphasia affect the carer and their relationship with the person with aphasia? *Aphasiology, 28*(11), 1301–1319. https://doi.org/10.1080/02687038.2014.928665

9

Loneliness in Chronic Illness Care: Health and Community Care Professional Perspectives

Health professionals increasingly encounter patients whose chronic conditions are compounded by loneliness. As discussed in Chapter One, rising numbers of lonely patients seeking healthcare services and increased healthcare consultations may indicate insufficient community and social supports for individuals experiencing loneliness. For those with chronic illness and who are also lonely, their family doctor may be the only support option available to them (Jovicic & McPherson, 2020). This places health and community care professionals in the challenging position of increasingly needing to support patients experiencing loneliness, while simultaneously facing numerous challenges in doing so, including limited training, time constraints and healthcare systems designed primarily around medical rather than social needs.

Historically, healthcare systems have been structured to attend to acute rather than chronic issues. Accordingly, health and community care professionals have been trained primarily in medical models that seek to diagnose, treat and cure. More recently, it has been recognised that chronic illness comprises social and personal dimensions as well as clinical, which need to be addressed to enable people to manage and live well with their conditions. Yet, healthcare systems remain designed to

S. Lewis et al., *Unravelling the Layers of Chronic Illness and Loneliness*, https://doi.org/10.1007/978-981-96-7909-6_9

focus on and treat clinical signs and symptoms, so there is little space to explore the complex social and emotional aspects of illness, such as loneliness. These less tangible dimensions of the chronic illness experience are thus likely to be overlooked or under-recognised within healthcare systems optimised for measurable clinical outcomes. There is now extensive research showing that healthcare encounters for chronic illness management are overwhelmingly weighted towards medication adherence and lifestyle changes (e.g. diet and physical activity) (Chelby et al., 2023; Franklin et al., 2019, 2021; Hughes et al., 2019), while "non-medical" issues such as loneliness are viewed by patients and healthcare professionals alike as secondary topics for discussion in medical encounters (Kharicha et al., 2017; Park et al., 2020), or, as discussed in Chapter One, deemed a matter of individual responsibility for the individual to address alone.

A further challenge surrounds the identification of loneliness in healthcare encounters. As discussed in Chapter One, in clinical settings loneliness is neither treated as a disease nor a psychiatric illness and there is evidence that loneliness is routinely missed in medical encounters with patients with chronic illnesses (Franklin et al., 2019). In the clinical literature (Galvez-Hernandez et al., 2022; Smith et al., 2024), health and community care professionals are increasingly being called on to screen for loneliness, as they do for other risk factors such as smoking and alcohol use. Also as discussed in Chapter One, standardised measurement tools (e.g. the UCLA Loneliness Scale by Russell et al., 1980) are promoted, rather than identification of loneliness through exploring patients' perspectives and experiences (Perissinotto et al., 2012).

There is also the related challenge of providing appropriate and adequate support to lonely patients. Health and community care professionals report that they have a limited array of solutions at their disposal to respond to loneliness. Unsurprisingly, they report feeling uncertain or constrained in how to alleviate loneliness due to a lack of skills, time, and options to do so (Van de Zwet et al., 2009). Thus, greater clarity is needed on what health and care professionals can do, and should be expected to do, to address the complex interplay of loneliness and chronic illness (Jovicic & McPherson, 2020). Insights from health and community care professionals who are supporting lonely patients are important in ensuring that future policies and interventions are grounded in real-world practice, ensuring that policies for loneliness in chronic condition care have practical application and are informed by the realities and complexities of health and community care delivery.

In this chapter, we explore the experiences of health and community care professionals who support and care for people with chronic illness who are experiencing loneliness. Below we draw on data from interviews with a diverse group of health and community care professionals (See Table 3 in Appendix) to analyse the complexities and challenges they experienced in conceptualising, identifying and responding to loneliness in their patients with chronic illnesses.

Defining Loneliness

Interviews with health and community care professionals show that, consistent with the literature, they view loneliness as being multidimensional, layered, hard to define and difficult to delineate from social isolation, distress or lack of social support (Courtin & Knapp, 2017; Jovicic & McPherson, 2020; Mansfield et al., 2021). Some participants indicated that they had not given much thought to how loneliness differed from social isolation. Professionals' conceptions of loneliness ranged from normalising it as being "part of the human experience" to the product of weakening social bonds or interpersonal disruption such as "feeling disconnected from social supports" or "feeling disconnected from normal social interaction". Similar to our participants with chronic illness (as discussed in Chapter Two), they also reported that, for people with chronic illness, loneliness is associated with feeling "misunderstood", "worthless", "like an outcast", or struggling "for validation" of their illness. The experience of loneliness was also likened to feeling "very empty", like "quality of life is depleted", like being in a "dark hole", and the absence of intimacy and care:

> They feel lonely because they don't feel that anyone understands that they're not getting supported. (Isla, registered nurse, community setting).

Some participants, like Georgia, a registered nurse working in general practice, were critical of binary understandings of loneliness, suggesting that loneliness and social isolation had "different levels":

> I think they're just on different levels. Connecting with someone socially is that shared interest, which can help a bit, but people can then go home. And some people are quite self-resilient. They can live happily alone. But I think we're social beings and a lot of people prefer to live with someone or knowing someone's there. But it could be that it's a pet. (Georgia, 50s, nurse, general practice)

Illustrating the multiple layers of loneliness, a medical specialist working in a public hospital, described how loneliness can emanate from a lack of intimacy and warmth across multiple kinds of relationships—with health professionals, intimate partners, friends and acquaintances:

> If someone senses a lack or an insufficiency in what they consider that they would like or they would need in terms of intimacy or trust or warmth or safety or caring then that may well be identified or named as loneliness. (Edward, 50s, medical specialist, public hospital setting)

Participants also described loneliness as the absence of meaningful pursuits or lack of purpose: "They used to have a whole life" (Jane, 40 s, social worker, community setting); "they don't feel that they can do things that actually bring meaning to their life" (Isla, registered nurse, community setting). While professionals said that they were aware that some of their patients were likely to be lonely, many (especially those working in clinical settings) had not given much thought to this issue in their everyday professional practice. A community pharmacist described an awareness of the presence of loneliness but indicated it was something that stayed at the margins of their interactions with their patients, attributing this partly to their professional socialisation and training:

> It's probably not something that I have thought about, other than—I mean, I guess you're probably peripherally sensitised to it because you know that there is something there, but it hasn't been brought out into the open… I mean, [loneliness] is peripheral, isn't it? If you're a

> practitioner, you've got a practitioner mindset. (Ian, 50s, pharmacist, community setting)

Recognising and Talking About Loneliness

When asked how they identified if a patient was lonely, health and community care professionals said that it was rarely something they or their patients brought up directly. As Isla noted:

> I don't know if I actually say, "Do you feel lonely?" Yeah, I guess it's something I very much gauge from their conversation from, again, their pointers. And I think it's fairly obvious perhaps for some. And some people do volunteer that information. Yeah, maybe once in a while I might, but I guess I don't always actually come out with the words, "Do you feel lonely?" I guess the depression and anxiety perhaps comes out more. People will offer that more. (Isla, registered nurse, community setting).

> I probably wouldn't ask that upfront either. I would assume, but they wouldn't state that they're lonely, yeah. They would say they don't have much contact. They spend a lot of time on their own, that's what they say. (Pamela, 50s, community worker, community setting)

Many commented that patients' hesitancy to bring up loneliness was likely associated with loneliness being a sensitive and potentially stigmatising issue. As Michelle said:

> These are hard things to talk about and people don't want to and there is a lot of shame and stigma attached to saying, "oh, I feel lonely." (Michelle, 30s, registered nurse, public hospital setting).

Other participants discussed how patients' fear of losing their independence or "being removed from their home" was another strong driver for patients to avoid admitting that they were struggling with loneliness. As a way around this, they described the need to identify loneliness "in a non-threatening way":

> …they do not want anybody else to find out because they're very comfortable managing in their own environment. But they're worried, "If I open the door, somebody's going to figure out how I live and how my house looks like and that means that I'm going to lose my independence." And so, therefore they want to live alone, disconnect from the social circles and things for that reason. So, there's many, many reasons. Sometimes it's more of being aware what is happening and then trying to identify it in a non-threatening way. (Rupert, medical specialist, public hospital setting)

For these reasons, professionals described the need to pick up on "clues", "vibes", or "subtle non-verbal cues'" that alluded to the person being lonely or that signalled to the professional the need to "dig deeper". These signals included the person talking "around the issue", struggling with self-care of their chronic illness, referring to their anxiety or depression, lack of sleep, having low motivation or flat affect, or saying that they have no one to provide care or support, as described by a community nurse and diabetes nurse educator:

> People don't come in and say, "I'm lonely." People come in and say, "I'm not sleeping," or "I don't feel as motivated as I used to." Nine times out of 10, we all know it starts with the physiological signs. "I've got pain. I've got this" (Rosanna, 60s, nurse, community setting).

> Because when I'm talking about diabetic self-care, and then the same story happens…they're not checking their sugar level at home, and then when we dig deeper into it and they will say… Like, "I don't care anymore," and that's not what's good for them. Or they'll become miserable and don't feel having energy to do things for themselves. (Erin, 60s, diabetes nurse educator)

As indicated above, professionals rarely used the word "lonely" in their conversations with their patients. They considered loneliness a sensitive topic and, cognisant of not wanting to provoke shame or distress, actively sought to avoid potentially stigmatising language by using indirect language and open questions about what activities the person did, who was in their network, or their employment status, as proxies for (risk of) loneliness:

> I do say to them, "Do you like to be social? Would you like to be social more?" (Bettina, 40s, disability services coordinator, community setting)
> We ask, "Have you got good supports or has your support network changed lately or have you changed in employment, change in family, change in marital status, change in...?" (Robert, 50s, paramedic, public hospital setting)

This approach was viewed by professionals as a less stigmatising and more caring way to explore loneliness with the patient. This is illustrated by Candice, who described the value of feeling comfortable opening conversations with their patients about loneliness, through being curious about the person's life and showing that they were invested in helping them:

> I do like to talk to my patients, and sometimes they would straight away tell you that, "I want to go home" or "I miss my family." Sometimes if they don't tell you straight away, you can gauge their emotional situation by the way they look. So whether they look composed or whether they look content or whether they look down, low mood, not engaging, not making eye contact, only answering yes or no without speaking much further. Most of the time... when I put myself as someone who wants to help them, interested in them, wants to advocate for them, they will open up and they will tell me that they're lonely. (Candice, registered nurse, hospital and community setting).

Unlike many other participants, Candice discussed the value of asking questions openly:

> I'm comfortable doing it [asking about loneliness]. I do ask questions quite openly. Almost all the time they would reply and they'll just tell me. Yeah, so I find that as long as I ask, they will answer. (Candice, registered nurse, hospital and community setting)

Candice's comfort with open discussion was in contrast to most participants' experiences. While acknowledging that loneliness had a significant impact on chronic illness, many professionals described feeling uncomfortable engaging with this issue as it fell outside of "the normal parameters" of their role or they did not feel well-equipped to meaningfully respond. Nonetheless, they still felt the weight of responsibility to "provide advice" or "solve" the problem of loneliness. This notion of responsibility, coupled with a sense of helplessness about what to do to "fix" loneliness, was a significant obstacle for professionals in beginning a dialogue about loneliness, as exemplified by a community pharmacist:

> Every pharmacist or GP has their patients that you see a lot and they have problems, that they're not within the normal parameters and [not] easy to fix. And practitioners like to feel like they can fix things. So if you can't fix it, then you feel a bit powerless and there's the uncertainty involved in talking to someone if you can't give them a solution. (Ian, 50s, pharmacist, community setting)

Strategies for Supporting Lonely Patients

Professionals who engaged with the issue of loneliness with their patients employed a range of different strategies to support these patients. These strategies were contingent on the settings and professions in which they were working, as well as the cohort of patients that they engaged with. Some professionals said that they encouraged their patients to talk with their GP. They saw the GP as playing a key role in being able to support people who are lonely, as they could refer them to relevant community services or other professionals, such as social workers or psychologists:

> We can often give information, but we can't obviously action it in terms of referrals. So, it's important that they have a good connection with their GP, and we would encourage them to talk about loneliness with them and see about making further connections from there. (Isla, registered nurse, community setting)

> Sometimes it's the social worker, sometimes it will be the psychology services, which we do not have in our services, so then we would have to access either through the GP or through other community-based services. (Rupert, medical specialist, public hospital setting)

Another strategy that professionals used in supporting patients who were lonely involved focusing on nurturing the patient/professional relationship, through acknowledging, validating or normalising the patient's experience of loneliness. Professionals did this by being "present", using touch, a smile, or "having a giggle", asking people "how they are and what support they need", and checking in with people who are lonely with a phone call, email or text message. Highlighting how they used these strategies, Candice said:

> Just your presence, being with them, makes a big difference. A lot of the time touch, if appropriate, I find is very meaningful as well. Be available. Just smile and say, "how are you? Can I do anything for you?" and be there for them. Be available to listen. (Candice, registered nurse, hospital and community setting)

Similarly, Kevin, a physiotherapist working in private practice, commented about the importance of validating people's experiences of loneliness, rather than providing a solution:

> I think, for some of them, it's having someone hear their concerns and issues. Most of the time I don't provide any solutions. I listen. One in particular finds it really, really helpful...so it could be this person might be doing their rehab exercise, plus they're talking about things that are bothering them. So, it's probably a dual therapy, in a way. It's talking therapy, plus the exercise. So, I think that that's probably a good thing. (Kevin, 50s, physiotherapist, private practice)

Support groups also featured prominently in professionals' accounts of supporting people living with chronic illness who are lonely. Professionals commented that participating in a support group provides people with an opportunity to be present with others, and to have their experiences heard and understood by others with similar experiences. For example, Derinda described support groups as providing people with a supportive, empowering and motivating environment:

> A lot of the time they've come to our clinic and they've been through a lot of the health system and what we hear is that they feel they haven't

> been listened to and they haven't been understood and they haven't been validated. So, when they can come to a group environment and start to share what their experience is and the person next to them can say, "I understand what you're going through," that's really empowering because they're no longer the only person that's going through it. (Derinda, 50s, physiotherapist, public hospital setting)

However, other professionals emphasised that joining a support group can be difficult for people experiencing loneliness and that the timing needed to be right for when to introduce them to a group. Reflecting on the importance of timing and fostering a sense of autonomy and support for people to travel their own path, in their own time, Rosanna, a community nurse and Sarah, a GP, commented:

> When people are feeling isolated, they don't really want to be pushed into a social recreation group or basket weaving, whatever group you think might help. … I think what they want to do is actually call it that in their own space, give it a name, recognise it, and then work through it. (Rosanna, 60s, nurse, community setting)

> I tell people about them [support groups] when it's appropriate, tell people that these things exist. My experience has been when you try and push it too hard you actually just get them to go once and they don't keep going anyway. (Sarah, 60s, GP, general practice)

Other strategies that professionals described using to support people experiencing loneliness included encouraging people to reconnect with friends, to engage in low-demand activities such as watching movies, art and working on relationships in their home environment. They also described encouraging patients to engage in exercise or sporting, leisure or social groups. Not only was this to foster social connectedness, but was an aspect of self-management. Here, the focus was on supporting people to have the tools, skills, motivation and confidence to manage their social lives and their illness:

> So I guess what we're trying to do is to teach them the tools to self-manage and re-engage with life, and hopefully part of that is their

> social part of their life as well. So yeah, that's huge. (Derinda, 50s, physiotherapist, public hospital)

Feeling Powerless in the System

Professionals also discussed the many system-wide barriers that impeded their capacity to meaningfully support people living with chronic illness who are lonely. Challenges often related to time constraints. However, they also stemmed from the fragmentation and complexities within and across sectors, funding structures, and a lack of suitable options available to help ameliorate loneliness. As Sarah, a GP said:

> [Loneliness] increases the consultation time. Most of my patients ... don't have any money. But that's a cost of practice and cost to me personally. It also increases our nursing time. I have a limited number of new patients, basically because I am so busy with the complexity of my patients... The billing structure is designed that you just see a patient quickly and get them out and then you actually will, theoretically, make some money (Sarah, 60s, GP, general practice)

While professionals spoke of a shortage of mainstream services, they also highlighted that the organisations providing support each have different priorities and eligibility requirements, often time-limited funding, and these factors complicate care coordination:

> I don't know what local [services], if there are any more, I mean, there may well be, that I could link people in with, I suppose. Or sometimes you think you've found one and then it just doesn't fit. There's all the certain eligibility criteria and that sort of thing. (Michelle, 30s, registered nurse, public hospital setting)

> Resources are sort of fragmented and hard to fit the right person at the right stage in the right group...it depends on where they live, on transport, on all sorts of things. (Kevin, 50s, physiotherapist, private practice)

Participants also highlighted broader funding issues such as those related to housing and transport. For example, Jane, a social worker working in the community sector, spoke of the struggles patients experienced in accessing funding for transport that supports a holistic approach to care. Highlighting how subsidised transport is limited to supporting people's medical rather than social needs, Jane commented:

> If you can't drive, you'll get transport to and from appointments, and that's it. So, anything outside of attending your medical appointments, if you're not able to drive or have someone to drive, getting transport out of your house, if you can't walk, is incredibly difficult.... Oh, absolutely, if there was a magic pill for transport, it would make life a lot easier. (Jane, 40s, social worker, community setting)

Pamela spoke of the lack of case management support needed to address the recursive nature of chronic illness and loneliness for people in complex circumstances:

> There's classic conditions of them becoming isolated due to inability to recover, crippling pain, and then the mental health. They become really lonely, a lot of them will push family away, there's marriage breakup, relationship breakup, isolation from kids through marriage breakup.... They really are so unwell that they can't function themselves. And there's a big chronic gap for that I guess, one-on-one type advocacy support, old-fashioned style case management role, where you're actually helping them to do a lot of basic stuff. (Pamela, 50s, community worker, community setting)

In a few instances, professionals discussed ways in which they went beyond the confines of their role or the setting in which they worked to meet the needs of people experiencing loneliness. For example, Robert described taking a lonely person to the hospital, even though ambulance services are usually for physical and life-threatening emergencies:

> Ambulance services generally, we're really trying to look for risks of injuries falls, are they coping, are they going to survive the night sort of attitude. We wouldn't generally transport someone if we thought they

> were at risk of being lonely, which is a bit of a shame. But sometimes when we realise, there's not really a question, "Are you lonely? You better come to hospital." Sometimes the symptoms don't seem that bad but they probably could do with some contact and maybe we'll get them in contact with the social worker or one of the nurses. (Robert, 50s, paramedic, public hospital setting)

Robert went on to say: "If we can help facilitate that, excellent, we've been the conduit to help, to get the ball rolling".

The pressure to explore various avenues for connection and support for patients, along with managing workload, budgets, and professional identity within the current system, can leave professionals feeling overwhelmed and underequipped. Many reported a sense of failure and despair at not being able to provide the care they perceived lonely people living with chronic illness need. This led some to question whether they were providing "good" care. Reflecting on the limits of what they can do, Robert commented:

> It can be very despairing. I just feel, you see someone that's really like quite isolated and obviously lonely. Sometimes we just, through our time pressures, we can't get involved. Yeah, it's terrible. (Robert, 50s, paramedic, public hospital setting)

Professionals described the complexity of trying to put in place "good care"' strategies while at the same time managing their own feelings of worry for patients. Exemplifying this issue, Pamela, a community worker working in rehabilitation, stated:

> It's difficult when the conversation of loneliness is also accompanied by the suicidal ideation. You do take on a level of worry about that person and their resilience and you try and put other strategies in place to do a wellbeing plan and make sure your bases are covered. But yeah, it's hard, because you still have your own feelings around that and your own empathy. For me, that's hard to see. (Pamela, 50s, community worker, community setting)

Overall, professionals expressed a desire for adequate support and supervision to help them handle the emotional intensity of supporting people living with chronic illness and loneliness. Many called for information on community services, mental health training, and strategies for sensitive conversations. A few expressed the need for specific guidelines and training on recognising and engaging with the topic of loneliness, suggesting that loneliness be a topic discussed in multidisciplinary meetings. Speaking of the benefits of guidelines Rupert stated:

> I think having proper guidelines for everybody to utilise, at least a framework, starting with what are the flags to watch out for when you're assessing a patient, because then at least that flag will raise a conversation. And then once you recognise it, then you need the staff to be trained in how to engage with these patients. (Rupert, medical specialist, public hospital setting)

Conclusion

Our research shows that within health and community care encounters, loneliness often remains unspoken and unacknowledged. This finding adds further weight to the importance of addressing the stigma and shame that surrounds loneliness (Neves & Petersen, 2025). Yet, stigma of loneliness was only part of the reticence to talk about loneliness in clinical encounters. Feeling powerless to "fix" the problem was featured prominently in participants' accounts. Although professionals expressed a sense of duty to help their lonely patients, they also reported difficulties in knowing how to respond to the problem in a system not well-equipped to support patients' social needs (Franklin et al., 2021). Thus, many of the strategies they drew on reflected the dominant individualistic approach discussed in earlier chapters. These strategies focused on equipping the patient to address their loneliness through joining support groups, engaging in activities and connecting with others. At the same time, professionals were aware that the institutional structures and systems they operated within, such as billing structures and time-limited appointments, along with fragmented or siloed health and social care systems challenged their capacity to do more than this.

Participants' accounts draw attention to the extra emotional and navigational labour associated with supporting patients who are experiencing loneliness in addition to multiple chronic physical and mental health conditions. The challenges articulated by participants highlight the need for more supportive infrastructures to mitigate the emotional impact on professionals and support the well-being of professionals and patients alike. Professionals identified the need for training, ongoing support and infrastructure that attend to the specificities and complexities of supporting people with chronic illnesses and loneliness. They also pointed to the vital importance of situating care in the social context of patients. Importantly, developing new approaches to care that can address social factors such as loneliness along with, for many patients, multiple chronic conditions also requires a better understanding of what constitutes "good" care in this context (Mol, 2008).

Our findings add weight to the importance of shifting away from approaches to loneliness which focus on the individual, towards approaches that embrace collaborative and collective care practices, in meaningfully supporting people with chronic illness experiencing loneliness. As discussed in Chapter One, systems built around the medical model and acute care, tend to marginalise the intricate social aspects of living with chronic illnesses and the changes needed to address social dimensions of chronic illness such as loneliness While there is widespread acknowledgement at the policy level that approaches to chronic condition care must be person-centred, community-informed, and attend to social issues like loneliness, these findings and those of others (see also Franklin et al., 2019, 2021; Raus et al., 2020) indicate that their application in real-world practice is difficult. At the same time, placing responsibility for addressing loneliness within healthcare systems risks both medicalising social problems and diverting attention and resources from the community sectors that may be better equipped to tackle loneliness. While health professionals play an important role in recognising loneliness, these findings highlight the limits of expecting healthcare systems to address what is fundamentally a social issue.

References

Chelby, N., Smith, J., & Brown, L. (2023). The impact of chronic conditions on quality of life: A comprehensive review. *Journal of Chronic Disease Management, 15*(2), 123–145.

Courtin, E., & Knapp, M. (2017). Social isolation, loneliness and health in old age: A scoping review. *Health & Social Care in the Community, 25*(3), 799–812.

Franklin, M., Lewis, S., Willis, K., Rogers, A., Venville, A., & Smith, L. (2019). Goals for living with a chronic condition: The relevance of temporalities, dispositions, and resources. *Social Science & Medicine, 233*, 13–20.

Franklin, M., Willis, K., Lewis, S., Rogers, A., & Smith, L. (2021). Between knowing and doing person-centredness: A qualitative examination of health professionals' perceptions of roles in self-management support. *Health, 25*(3), 339–356.

Galvez-Hernandez, P., González-de Paz, L., & Muntaner, C. (2022). Primary care-based interventions addressing social isolation and loneliness in older people: A scoping review. *British Medical Journal Open, 12*(2), Article e057729.

Hughes, S., Lewis, S., Willis, K., Rogers, A., Wyke, S., & Smith, L. (2019). Goal setting in group programmes for long-term condition self-management support: Experiences of patients and healthcare professionals. *Psychology & Health, 35*(1), 70–86. https://doi.org/10.1080/08870446.2019.1623891

Jovicic, A., & McPherson, S. (2020). To support and not to cure: General practitioner management of loneliness. *Health & Social Care in the Community, 28*(2), 376–384.

Kharicha, K., Illife, S., Manthorpe, J., Chew-Graham, C. A., Cattan, M., Goodman, C., & Walters, K. (2017). What do older people experiencing loneliness think about primary care or community based interventions to reduce loneliness? A qualitative study in England. *Health & Social Care in the Community, 25*(6), 1733–1742. https://doi.org/10.1111/hsc.12438

Mansfield, L., Victor, C., Meads, C., Daykin, N., Tomlinson, A., Lane, J., & Golding, A. (2021). A conceptual review of loneliness in adults: Qualitative evidence synthesis. *International Journal of Environmental Research and Public Health, 18*(21), 11522.

Mol, A. (2008). The logic of care: Health and the problem of patient choice. Routledge.

Neves, B. B., & Petersen, A. (2025). The social stigma of loneliness: A sociological approach to understanding the experiences of older people. *The Sociological Review, 73*(2), 362–383.

Park, S., Lee, S., & Kim, J. (2020). Understanding the perception of non-medical issues in healthcare encounters: A qualitative study. *Journal of Health Communication, 25*(3), 123–134.

Perissinotto, C. M., Cenzer, I. S., & Covinsky, K. E. (2012). Loneliness in older persons: A predictor of functional decline and death. *Archives of Internal Medicine, 172*(14), 1078–1084.

Raus, K., Mortier, E., & Eeckloo, K. (2020). Challenges in turning a great idea into great health policy: The case of integrated care. *BMC Health Services Research, 20*, 1–9.

Russell, D., Peplau, L. A., & Cutrona, C. E. (1980). The revised UCLA loneliness scale: Concurrent and discriminant validity evidence. *Journal of Personality and Social Psychology, 39*(3), 472–480.

Smith, S., Lally, P., Steptoe, A., Chavez-Ugalde, Y., Beeken, R. J., & Fisher, A. (2024). Prevalence of loneliness and associations with health behaviours and body mass index in 5835 people living with and beyond cancer: A cross-sectional study. *BMC Public Health*. https://doi.org/10.1186/s12889-024-17797-3

Van der Zwet, J., Koelewijn-van Loon, M. S., & Van den Akker, M. (2009). Lonely patients in general practice: A call for revealing GPs' emotions? A qualitative study. *Family Practice, 26*(6), 501–509.

10

Reimagining Connection in Chronic Illness: Towards Inclusive Approaches to Loneliness

When we embarked on writing this book the public gaze on loneliness was intense, yet the personal stories of those who experienced it were largely silent and underacknowledged. Thus, one of our goals in this book, and the study it draws from, was to amplify the voices of people living with chronic illness and loneliness, make visible their experience of loneliness, in all its complexity, and learn from them about how they could be supported.

Recognising the value of giving space for people to express their experiences of loneliness and illness in-depth and in their own words, we start this concluding chapter by sharing final reflections offered by participants at the end of their interviews or in correspondence to us after their interviews. These quotes illustrate the positive impact of listening, without offering advice or remedy, or imposing a particular understanding of what loneliness means or how it is experienced, in feeling seen and recognised.

> I saw the story, Karen's story in our local paper, and it just really resonated with me. I looked at it and I thought, "That's an article about me." And I wanted to put myself out there and be involved and talk about the stuff that I don't usually talk about, because I know there are so many

S. Lewis et al., *Unravelling the Layers of Chronic Illness and Loneliness*, https://doi.org/10.1007/978-981-96-7909-6_10

> people out there like me, but we're all hidden away and not talking about it. (Michella, during her first interview)

> Yeah, funnily enough I'm feeling better than I was before the call. Just because I talk about it so rarely, I really was interested in the opportunity to tell my story. Sometimes I just feel like I don't exist and that my experiences just don't matter or make any mark on this existence. I think it's something that I wanted to do. As soon as I saw it, I really felt that calling that I wanted to participate in this study and continue to broaden the understanding of loneliness and chronic disease. Because it's different for everyone, it's really complex, and more healthcare professionals need to be trained in that area. (Freya, when asked how she was feeling after the interview)

> Thank you very much. It's been good. I've enjoyed every minute of it. Thank you for listening to me. (Rosemary, during her third interview)

> Thank you for caring enough to conduct this study. People like you give me hope. I am glad I had the opportunity to participate. You made me feel heard and were very considerate, inquisitive and kind. (Tina, email after receiving a participant summary of results)

Like other research which has shown the positive effects of participating in qualitative research (Grace et al., 2016; Hutchinson et al., 1994), some participants said the opportunity to talk about loneliness in the safe space of the interview was cathartic, restorative or remedial as it enabled them to give voice to, and reflect on, a previously hidden or unspeakable topic.

> I'm feeling good about it. I'm feeling like that last thing I just said then was probably more of me feeling like my loneliness isn't that abnormal and it isn't that huge. It's not minimising it for me, but it's normalising it more. (Rory, when asked how they were feeling at the end of the interview)

> Just talking to you, it's always insightful talking to people because it forces you to look inside a bit and to pull out things from cupboards that you have closed. It makes you look at things. (Greg, during his interview)

> I actually slept the whole night through, the wonders of an interesting conversation. (Greg, email the day after the interview)

> I feel nice. It's been refreshing. It's reminded me so many things that are quite good. Yeah, I feel good. (Emma, when asked how she was feeling at the end of the interview)

> Well actually, it makes me feel better having a cry. It sounds silly, but now I've had a cry, it makes me feel better. Sometimes you can keep it there and it's all right. But when you have to actually verbalise it, then you start bawling. Thank you so much for your time, darling. (Ida, when asked how she was feeling at the end of the interview)

> A bit exhausted, but it's been nice to talk.... Probably a little bit difficult, but sometimes it helps to talk. And you don't talk about it a lot. I don't talk about it a lot, I suppose. But yeah. (Bernadette, when asked how she was feeling at the end of the interview)

> It's very thought provoking. It gets me thinking. (Rob, in response to being asked if there is anything else he wanted to share)

> I feel good. I feel good that I just got some of that stuff off my chest, I guess. (Tina, when asked how she was feeling at the end of the interview)

> That was great... I feel quite nice. (Tammy, at the end of her second interview)

Sharing and reflecting on their experiences could also be a catalyst for positive social changes.

> ...doing this kind of introspection and extrospection about yourself and others and that dynamic and flow, that's the critical part about the social connection, is it's not just you in it. It's about your relationship with others. And so yeah, I think I would definitely love to [do another interview]. I'm sure I'll think of some more things and have these conversations. I'd love to do another interview and see what I discover from other people and how they think or feel. Again, crystallise more what I might like then on the basis of what other people... a month or two

would be great. Give me time to play around with these things. (Astrid, after her first interview)

I really appreciate the opportunity to talk through that with you and to engage in those kinds of reflections, because I still felt a bit raw about the weekend. And I think that, yeah, it's just something I can have a bit of a think about and put some other strategies in place. (Freya, during her second interview)

Some of it helps me too in sort of going through it and what I'm feeling or what I'm thinking. And yeah, I'm a lot more in tune with things these days, than I used to be. And I think that comes with a lot of maturity and probably a lot of therapy as well, that I am getting a lot more understanding of my own needs and I can read myself a lot more as well. And I'd love to do your job. I love hearing other people's stories. I just love hearing about people's lives and things like that. It's been a really interesting conversation. Thank you for that. (Laura, at the end of her first interview)

In their follow-up interviews, some participants had taken steps to remediate their loneliness or described coming to a deeper "knowing" of self, that helped them think differently about what was possible for their future.

I found that I was relieved to get an awful lot that I was sort of hiding deep down in my cognition, without mentioning it to anybody, because there was nobody to mention it to. And so, I found that the fact of talking and being able to be so open, and as our conversation went on, I found that I was becoming more free to open up more… it was amazing how psychologically freeing it was. So, I was able to look at things in a different way, in a better, more inclusive way, rather than an exclusive way. Yes. I enjoyed that. […] After talking with you and reflecting on things, I began to realise that I had to do some active emotional, mental health work on changing my, not so much my beliefs, but my understanding of myself and where I was at. So I found it very useful, actually. Thank you. (Adelaide, during her third interview)

> Last time we spoke… that process of reflection started, and, as a result, I changed things. So, I think your piece of research is really interesting in that, not only does it observe something, but it changes it through the process of observation… I reflected on what was important to me. (Betty, during her third interview)

> The thing I gained most from your research was the opportunity to reflect and the changes I made as a result. I'm still working on those goals and my healing journey. (Betty, email after receiving a participant summary of results)

Talking while walking also had value (Kinney, 2017), not only in facilitating conversations about loneliness, but in fostering belonging within their community.

> It [was] lovely to go out and about like we did, feel part of something bigger. I'm taking my own advice—doing one thing a day; going to the gym; knowing that this will pass… Thank you for the kick into reflection. Don't like it much, but it is necessary. (Verna, email after her walking interview)

Listening, Not Fixing

As discussed in Chapters Four, Eight, and Nine, people with chronic illness, family members and other carers, and health and community care professionals, often struggle with how to talk about loneliness in their relationships due to shame, stigma, discomfort, indifference or lack of understanding. And yet, their stories also reveal the value in sharing experiences of loneliness and other social aspects of living with chronic illness. Giving space to share experiences and be heard can have utility, alongside broader socio-structural change, in informing how loneliness can be tackled at the level of micro-social interaction. For example, these insights can inform the development of discussion guides for health professionals about how they have conversations with people about loneliness, or how family members and friends can offer meaningful support.

Recognition and Authentic Relating

Opportunities to express oneself with authenticity, feeling known for one's "true" self and not being reduced to an illness- or carer-identity, feeling that one has social value, and recognition of the complexities of managing illness all fostered connectedness. As shown in Chapters Two and Eight, when experiences of illness or the work of care were overlooked, diminished or misunderstood by others, illness was a lonely and segregating experience (see also Lewis et al., 2024). The loneliness associated with misrecognition (i.e. the failure to adequately recognise the person for their true personhood) was most acutely felt by those with multiple, contested, and/or invisible illnesses; indicating that the nature of the illness and its legibility to others is important in shaping how loneliness is experienced and its effects. Responding to loneliness must therefore attend to the complexities of how chronic illness is constructed and lived (Manderson & Smith-Morris, 2010). Additionally, the complexities of multiple chronic conditions and how they are mis/understood, mis/read, and un/seen hindered opportunities to forge collective identities and access social support from peers or others with illnesses. In thinking about new approaches to loneliness, a key question will be how collective identities and solidarities can be cultivated in the context of multiple chronicity.

Authentic relating encompassed not only mutual understanding, but also mutual care and reciprocity. Having opportunities to care for and help others, and feel cared for in return, as discussed in Chapter Four, were integral to connectedness. This illustrates the importance of valuing interdependency, mutuality and collective forms of relating, as well as challenging the high societal value placed on independence, if we are to foster social connectedness and ensure that people with chronic illness feel they can access the social supports they need (Prainsack, 2018).

Safe Spaces for Being

Being with others who could hold space for and accommodate illness without expectations for performance or active social engagement was important in embracing those with chronic illness into the social scene. Chapter Six and Seven illustrate that when symptoms of illness exclude a person from traditional activity-based social engagement, there is value in creating safe and inclusive spaces (online and offline), where the person does not feel pressure to perform or *do* social connection (e.g. through engaging in a social activity or joining a group), and where they can feel known, respected and part of the social landscape.

Increasing recognition that features of built and natural environments can contribute to and alleviate loneliness has given rise to loneliness interventions that encourage people to spend time in nature (e.g. "nature prescriptions") (Astell-Burt et al., 2022; Bower et al., 2023; Litt et al., 2024). Yet for these kinds of initiatives to succeed, it will be important to think about how equitable access for people with chronic illness can be promoted and how affinity to place, and meaningful interactions within place, can be fostered. Artificial attempts to create spaces for belonging often fail because they are not responsive to the needs of the person and what they value. Thus, creating inclusive spaces for presence, connection, and community building must be informed by the needs of the communities they serve and orientated around what matters to them. We must also consider how health and social care spaces can be redesigned to better meet the social needs of those with chronic illness who are lonely and create more socially inclusive communities for all.

Cultivating Multiple Avenues to Meaningful Connection

Relational understandings of loneliness see loneliness as emerging within multiple human and non-human relationships and interactions (rather than emanating from within individual bodies). As shown across the chapters in this book, approaches to alleviating loneliness must go beyond a one-dimensional focus on supporting human relationships.

Loneliness can be ameliorated through connection to meaningful places, animals, routines, and shared rituals, as well as through fostering a deeper connection to self through art, music and stories (Neves et al., 2019). These connections are especially important to those with chronic illness because they do not require the same performative work or self-presentation as many human interactions. They allow for different rhythms of interaction that can better accommodate the unpredictability of chronic illness, important for those who feel left behind by their peers (as discussed in Chapter Three). Understanding how people with chronic illness cultivate connections beyond human relationships is critical. Equally important is ensuring that these non-human bases for connections are recognised, valued and supported as part of a more expansive approach to loneliness (Franklin, 2009; Franklin & Tranter, 2021; May, 2011, 2013; Neves et al., 2024).

Locating Chronic Condition Care in the Social Domain

In preventing and ameliorating loneliness, more must be done to challenge the cultural ideals that still infuse chronic condition care frameworks, such as the ideal of the self-sufficient individual who takes responsibility for managing their health, care, and relationships. As we have illustrated, the societal ideal of individualistic pursuits of health and wellness can be isolating—both for people with illness and for carers. New approaches are needed which embed chronic condition care in the social domain (Lewis et al., 2022; Prainsack, 2018). As Neves et al. (2019) argue, at the healthcare system level there is a need to move beyond fleeting acknowledgements of the social dimensions of chronic illness towards accounting for, and meaningfully addressing, these social aspects in chronic condition care and support. This will require developing social infrastructures and systems that are flexible and responsive to the messiness of illness and the diverse ways that people find and create social connectedness. In developing new approaches to chronic illness support we must also consider support for family members and others who provide care and support to people with illness, who, as shown in Chapter Eight, can also feel alone and isolated.

Shifting Responsibilities for Loneliness: From "I" to "We" Approaches

As discussed in earlier chapters, loneliness is increasingly constructed, especially in illness contexts, with reference to a biomedical perspective—one consequence of which is taking loneliness out of the social domain and into healthcare systems. Constructing loneliness as a medical problem inevitably directs responsibility for fixing the "problem" onto individual patients and health professionals and can risk diverting funding and resources away from communities and into healthcare systems and spaces. A relational understanding of loneliness helps us to move beyond approaches that frame loneliness as a private concern or medical problem, towards more inclusive perspectives that recognise it as a shared responsibility. Our research highlights the importance of viewing the cultivation of social connectedness as collectively constituted, shared practices, rather than individual actions, and loneliness as collectively produced. As we have shown, loneliness is deeply embedded in social processes and structures, and this demands a move away from a focus on the individual, towards approaches that embrace collaborative and collective care practices, in meaningfully supporting people with chronic illness who are experiencing loneliness.

New approaches must also draw industry and government institutions into the frame of social responsibility, to ensure that our approaches are supported by broader infrastructures of care. Health and chronic illness organisations play a crucial role in constructing new affirmative narratives of chronic illnesses that acknowledge their complexities but also encompass positive representations of living *well* with illness. Creating bespoke support structures that accommodate various levels of ability, preferences of engagement, and social circumstances are also critical.

Making Loneliness and Chronic Illness Visible

Central to relational approaches to loneliness is recognising the importance of shifting how loneliness is understood, represented and discussed, both in personal interactions and broader social arenas. As we have shown, part of this work involves changing how we talk (or don't talk) about loneliness and illness. Another means of enhancing the visibility of loneliness and changing how it is understood is through creative and arts-based approaches. Radley and Bell (2007) have pointed to the "anchoring potential" of visual "works of illness" in providing entry points into the personal "worlds of illness", and in creating shifts in how illnesses are normatively mis/understood. Creative expressions (including artwork, music, theatre, dance, and poetry) can be one way to reimagine social connectedness with illness.

New Directions for Research and Policy

In this book, we have provided nuanced insights into how chronic illness and loneliness coalesce in ways that evade neat capture and solution. The more expansive social understandings of loneliness and its more-than-human bases that are provided in this book are helpful in moving beyond current deficit-based understandings that emphasise loneliness as deficiencies in social relationships (Franklin, 2009; Franklin et al., 2019; Neves et al., 2024). Future approaches to loneliness for those with chronic illness must be grounded in their lived experiences and social contexts. Strengths-based, user-led approaches are needed that centre the experiences, knowledges and assets of individuals and communities affected by loneliness, and recognise, value and cultivate diverse forms of meaningful connecting. The insights of our research have clear policy and practice implications for supporting loneliness in contexts of chronic illness. Loneliness is collectively produced and experienced through a constellation of social relations and practices, meaning current dominant framings through a lens of "cure" cannot fully attend to its multidimensional and evolving nature. It is thus not surprising that many of the programs and initiatives aimed at "fixing" loneliness (or perhaps more accurately fixing lonely individuals) in cohorts with chronic illness have had limited sustained success. Long-term data on program effectiveness remains limited and there is little understanding of how different illnesses require different approaches.

The path forward lies not in trying to "fix" loneliness in individuals but in building communities that create space for authentic connection across differences in health status and ability. Alternative relational approaches are needed that are grounded in what makes connection meaningful for those with chronic illness and that recognise how what counts as meaningful social connection varies across individuals, settings and illness types, and is cultivated in multiple ways. These approaches require building social infrastructures for inclusive communities while recognising that meaningfully responding to loneliness requires ongoing practices, care and support rather than one-time solutions. While new approaches must always centre the experiences and priorities of individuals, to ensure they are person-centred, they must also attend to social context including the social practices that help and hinder social connectedness (Ozawa-de Silva & Parsons, 2020). Looking ahead, addressing chronic illness and loneliness requires a multidisciplinary approach and action at multiple levels (micro, meso, and macro). This demands a fundamental reconceptualisation of how social institutions approach health and social connection. Such approaches require:

- Participatory approaches that centre lived experience of those affected by loneliness and chronic illness.
- Bringing together diverse stakeholders including policymakers, sociologists, anthropologists, urban planners, psychologists, and health practitioners.
- Learning from international examples of effective approaches, while developing locally appropriate responses. Cross-country comparisons could also illuminate how different institutional arrangements, and social structures shape the experience of loneliness in chronic illness.

- Infrastructure development that accommodates the unpredictable nature of chronic illness.
- Integration of creative approaches that can reshape public understanding and representation of chronic illness.

While all levels of government have provided varying degrees of support for loneliness programs, in Australia the lack of an overarching national loneliness framework leaves decision-makers with little guidance about where to direct resources, what approaches are likely to work and for whom. Moreover, addressing chronic illness and loneliness requires examining how multiple intersecting health and social systems, from health care to urban planning, can help or perpetuate existing inequalities. This includes consideration of how built and natural environments impact social connection and cohesion.

To create meaningful change, we must examine how loneliness stigma interplays with ableism in the daily lives of people with chronic illness; and raise public awareness through positive representations of living with chronic illness, while acknowledging its challenges. Success requires ensuring that social and material infrastructures support individuals and communities in cultivating social connectedness in ways that align with their needs, while simultaneously addressing the broader structural inequalities that shape experiences of both chronic illness and loneliness.

Moving away from prescriptive approaches and developing flexible, responsive systems that accommodate the messiness of illness, and the diverse ways people create connection will be essential. This requires a comprehensive suite of approaches that may include initiatives to strengthen social bonds and forge new connections on- and off-line, designing architectures that foster social connectivity, promoting connections with non-human beings, training and supporting our health and social care workforce in caring for loneliness, connecting people to meaningful work and valued social roles, and efforts to address loneliness stigma (Franklin & Tranter, 2021). Moving forward requires placing lived experience at the heart of all approaches, while also acknowledging that meaningfully responding to the complex mosaic of chronic illness and loneliness is fundamentally a matter of equity. Only by addressing the structural inequalities that leave people with chronic illness lonely and disconnected, can we ensure that we build inclusive communities that create opportunities for social connectedness for all.

References

Astell-Burt, T., Hartig, T., Putra, I. G. N. E., Walsan, R., Dendup, T., & Feng, X. (2022). Green space and loneliness: A systematic review with theoretical and methodological guidance for future research. *Science of the Total Environment, 847*, Article 157521.

Bower, M., Kent, J., Patulny, R., Green, O., McGrath, L., Teesson, L., & Rugel, E. (2023). The impact of the built environment on loneliness: A systematic review and narrative synthesis. *Health & Place, 79*, Article 102962.

Franklin, A. S. (2009). On loneliness. *Geografiska Annaler: Series b, Human Geography, 91*(4), 343–354.

Franklin, A., & Tranter, B. (2021). Loneliness and the cultural, spatial, temporal and generational bases of belonging. *Australian Journal of Psychology, 73*(1), 57–69.

Franklin, A., Barbosa Neves, B., Hookway, N., Patulny, R., Tranter, B., & Jaworski, K. (2019). Towards an understanding of loneliness among Australian men: Gender cultures, embodied expression and the social bases of belonging. *Journal of Sociology, 55*(1), 124–143.

Grace, D., Steinberg, M., Chown, S. A., Jollimore, J., Parry, R., & Gilbert, M. (2016). "It's almost therapeutic, right? Because it's almost like that session that I never had": Gay men's accounts of being a participant in HIV research. *AIDS Care, 28*(10), 1306–1311. https://doi.org/10.1080/09540121.2016.1178701

Hutchinson, S. A., Wilson, M. E., & Wilson, H. S. (1994). Benefits of participating in research interviews. *Image: the Journal of Nursing Scholarship, 26*(2), 161–166. https://doi.org/10.1111/j.1547-5069.1994.tb00937.x

Kinney, P. (2017). Walking interviews. *Social research update, 67*(1–4).

Lewis, S., Willis, K., Bismark, M., & Smallwood, N. (2022). A time for self-care? Frontline health workers' strategies for managing mental health during the COVID-19 pandemic. *SSM-Mental Health, 2*, Article 100053.

Lewis, S., Willis, K., Smith, L., Dubbin, L., Rogers, A., Lindegaard Moensted, M., & Smallwood, N. (2024). There but not really involved: The meanings of loneliness for people with chronic illness. *Social Science & Medicine, 343*, Article 116596. https://doi.org/10.1016/j.socscimed.2024.116596

Litt, J. S., Coll-Planas, L., Sachs, A. L., Rochau, U., Jansson, A., Dostálová, V., & Pitkälä, K. H. (2024). Nature-based social interventions for people experiencing loneliness: The rationale and overview of the RECETAS project. *Cities & Health, 8*(3), 418–431. https://doi.org/10.1080/23748834.2023.2300207

Manderson, L., & Smith-Morris, C. (Eds.). (2010). *Chronic conditions, fluid states: Chronicity and the anthropology of illness*. Rutgers University Press.

May, V. (2011). Self, belonging and social change. *Sociology, 45*(3), 363–378.

May, V. (2013). *Connecting self to society: Belonging in a changing world*. Bloomsbury Publishing.

Neves, B., Sanders, A., Warren, N., & Ko, P. C. (2024). Loneliness in later life as existential inequality. *Sociology, 58*(3), 659–681. https://doi.org/10.1177/00380385231208649

Neves, B. B., Sanders, A., & Kokanović, R. (2019). "It's the worst bloody feeling in the world": Experiences of loneliness and social isolation among older people living in care homes. *Journal of Aging Studies, 49*, 74–84.

Ozawa-de Silva, C., & Parsons, M. (2020). Toward an anthropology of loneliness. *Transcultural Psychiatry, 57*(5), 613–622.

Prainsack, B. (2018). The "we" in the "me" solidarity and health care in the era of personalized medicine. *Science, Technology, & Human Values, 43*(1), 21–44.

Radley, A., & Bell, S. E. (2007). Artworks, collective experience and claims for social justice: The case of women living with breast cancer. *Sociology of Health & Illness, 29*(3), 366–390.

Correction to: Unravelling the Layers of Chronic Illness and Loneliness

Correction to:
S. Lewis et al., *Unravelling the Layers of Chronic Illness and Loneliness*, https://doi.org/10.1007/978-981-96-7909-6

This book has been inadvertently published with an incorrect editor's order, which has now been corrected. The corrections to the cover and within the book have been updated with the changes.

The updated version of this book can be found at
https://doi.org/10.1007/978-981-96-7909-6

S. Lewis et al., *Unravelling the Layers of Chronic Illness and Loneliness*,
https://doi.org/10.1007/978-981-96-7909-6_11

Appendix

(See Tables for participant details A.1, A.2, A.3).

S. Lewis et al., *Unravelling the Layers of Chronic Illness and Loneliness*,
https://doi.org/10.1007/978-981-96-7909-6

Table A.1 Characteristics of participants with chronic illness and loneliness

Pseudonym	Age range	Living arrangement	Chronic illnesses
Adelaide	80s	Alone	Pulmonary fibrosis and osteoporosis
Astrid	30s	Family (siblings)	Asthma and anxiety
Bernadette	70s	Alone	Arthritis and depression
Betty	40s	Alone	Chronic pain, musculoskeletal issues and post-traumatic stress disorder
Bianca	60s	Alone	Fibromyalgia and severe food and chemical sensitivities
Bruno	30s	Parents	Chronic fatigue syndrome and anxiety
Cecilia	70s	Husband and dog	Complications after a lung transplant
Elizabeth*	30s	Alone with rabbits	Chronic bowel obstruction
Eloise	60s	Husband and dog	Rare neurological autoimmune condition, chronic leukemia and other chronic conditions
Emma	20s	Family (husband, child)	Diabetes and depression
Freya	40s	Alone	Endometriosis, chronic pain and post-traumatic stress disorder
Greg	60s	Alone with dog	Chronic back pain
Holly	60s	Family (husband, son, daughter in law, grandchild)	Urinary incontinence, chronic pain and anxiety
Ida	60s	Alone	Multiple sclerosis
Jasper	50s	Daughter	Epilepsy
Jesinta	Teens	Family (parents, brothers, cats)	Autoimmune encephalitis and depression
Jessica	60s	Husband and dog	Multiple sclerosis
Laura	50s	Alone	Arthritis and bipolar disorder
Lea	20s	Family (grandmother, aunt)	Polycystic ovary syndrome and anxiety
Lisa	70s	Husband	Chronic back pain

(continued)

Table A.1 (continued)

Pseudonym	Age range	Living arrangement	Chronic illnesses
Luke	60s	Alone with therapy dog	Visual impairment, chronic pain, and other chronic conditions
May	20s	Family (mother, sister)	Rare auto-inflammatory condition causing headaches, painful joints and ulcers
Michael	80s	Wife	Complications from double lung transplant
Michella	50s	Alone with cat	Systemic lupus erythematosus
Natalia	30s	Children	Rheumatoid arthritis, fibromyalgia, asthma, chronic migraines and other chronic conditions
Nelly	70s	Alone with cat	Chronic obstructive pulmonary disease
Nick	50s	Alone	HIV, depression and anxiety disorder
Nicola	30s	Alone with cat	Multiple sclerosis
Oliver	50s	Wife and daughter	Diabetes and schizophrenia
Phil	60s	Family (mother, dog)	Osteoporosis and schizophrenia
Renee	70s	Alone	Chronic obstructive pulmonary disease
Rob	40s	Family (wife, children)	Multiple sclerosis
Rory	50s	Alone with dogs	Fibromyalgia, chronic pain, and depression
Rosemary	60s	Husband and dog	Tick-borne disease and progressive gait disorder
Ross	60s	Partner	Arthritis and chronic back pain

(continued)

Table A.1 (continued)

Pseudonym	Age range	Living arrangement	Chronic illnesses
Tammy	40s	Husband and sons	Multiple sclerosis
Tina	30s	Partner	Fibromyalgia, post-traumatic stress disorder and irritable bowel syndrome
Toby	20s	Family (mother, cats)	Rare genetic condition causing weakness, fatigue and concentration difficulties
Verna	60s	Alone with cat	Multiple sclerosis
Zarah	20s	Family (mother, siblings, grandparents)	Multiple sclerosis and depression

*At second interview had moved in with partner and partner's family

Table A.2 Characteristics of carers

Pseudonym	Age range	Duration providing care	Relationship to person
Alice	50s	20 years	Caring for husband with multiple sclerosis and depression
Audrey	30s	23 years	Caring for husband, children and mother, all with multiple conditions
Charlotte	60s	5 years	Caring for partner with multiple chronic conditions including gastrointestinal problems and lymphatic system disorder
Cindy	50s	15 years	Caring for son with epilepsy and autism
Clara	20s	10 years	Caring for mother with type 2 diabetes and hypertension
Danielle	20s	2 years	Caring for mother with hypertension and Alzheimer's disease
Dorothy	60s	13 years	Caring for daughter with multiple sclerosis, autism and other chronic conditions
Elaine	30s	14 years	Caring for grandmother with diabetes, hypertension and heart failure; and friend with lupus, endometriosis, and mental health conditions
Ella	20s	10 years	Caring for brother with auditory neuropathy and attention deficit hyperactivity disorder
Elsie	70s	5 years	Caring for son with cancer
Esther	60s	5 years	Caring for child with multiple sclerosis
Gina	70s	51 years	Caring for daughter with multiple genetic conditions and schizophrenia

(continued)

Table A.2 (continued)

Pseudonym	Age range	Duration providing care	Relationship to person
Gloria	50s	37 years	Caring for children with multiple chronic mental and physical conditions
Henry	60s	2 years	Caring for daughter with anxiety disorder and autism
Jason	40s	7 years	Caring for children with anxiety disorder and autism
Josephine	30s	5 years	Caring for partner with multiple conditions
Juliet	20s	2 years	Caring for partner with fibromyalgia and polycystic ovary syndrome
Kara	30s	4 years	Caring for son with cystic fibrosis and pancreatic insufficiency
Larissa	50s	12 years	Caring for partner with chronic migraine
Miranda	30s	6 years	Caring for son with rare genetic condition and autism spectrum disorder
Molly	40s	20 years	Caring for partner with multiple sclerosis, anxiety and depression
Rachel	50s	4 years	Caring for son with schizophrenia
Rosalind	60s	3 years	Caring for ex-partner with spinal cord injury, diabetes, heart disease and chronic kidney disease
Sally	40s	11 years	Caring for daughter with a rare genetic condition
Victoria	30s	5 years	Caring for husband with lymphoma and post-transplant complications

(continued)

Table A.2 (continued)

Pseudonym	Age range	Duration providing care	Relationship to person
Vivian	50s	17 years	Caring for mother with diabetes and other chronic health conditions
Yvette	60s	30 years	Caring for daughter with chronic fatigue syndrome and movement disorder

Table A.3 Characteristics of health and community care professionals

Pseudonym	Age range	Role	Years experience	Setting
Amber	30s	Psychosexual Therapist	13	Community setting
Bernie	50s	Registered Nurse	18	Public
Bettina	40s	Disability Services Coordinator	1	Community setting
Candice	Unspecified	Registered Nurse	Unspecified	Public hospital and community setting
Carole	40s	Community Worker	10	Community setting
Derinda	50s	Physiotherapist	30	Public hospital
Edward	50s	Medical Specialist	30+	Public hospital
Erin	60s	Diabetes Nurse Educator	40+	Not specified
Georgia	50s	Registered Nurse	30	General practice
Heidi	40s	Disability Services Coordinator	3	Community setting
Ian	50s	Pharmacist	30	Community setting
Isla	Unspecified	Registered Nurse	16	Community setting
Jane	40s	Social Worker	8	Community setting
Kevin	50s	Physiotherapist	30	Private practice
Lyn	60s	Medical Specialist	30+	Private and public hospital
Maggie	40s	Paramedic	15	Public hospital
Mary	50s	Community Worker	2	Community setting
Michelle	30s	Registered Nurse	10	Public hospital

(continued)

Table A.3 (continued)

Pseudonym	Age range	Role	Years experience	Setting
Pamela	50s	Community Worker	23	Community setting
Robert	50s	Paramedic	30+	Public hospital
Rosanna	60s	Nurse	40+	Community setting
Rupert	Unspecified	Medical Specialist	Unspecified	Public hospital
Sarah	60s	General Practitioner	35+	General practice

FSC
www.fsc.org
MIX
Papier | Fördert
gute Waldnutzung
FSC® C083411

Kolibri 360 GmbH
Ferdinand-Jühlke-Straße 7
99095 Erfurt, Deutschland
produktsicherheit@kolibri360.de